COMING TO HARM REDUCTION KICKING AND SCREAMING:

SECOND EDITION

COMING TO HARM REDUCTION KICKING AND SCREAMING:

STORIES OF RADICALLY LOVING PEOPLE WHO USE DRUGS

SECOND EDITION

DEE-DEE STOUT. MA & JOE CLIFFORD. MFA

Square Tire Books

Austin, TX

Squaretirerecords.com

First published by Square Tire Books, 2025

ISBN: 978-1-960725-21-9

Library of Congress Control Number: 2025901315

DEDICATION

For Jessie, Kay & Nels and George & Lucile

My grandparents and original Harm Reductionists

who loved me unconditionally – and not perfectly - through it all.

...DDS

Dedicated to everyone who won't give up. Keep on fighting.

...JNC

TABLE OF CONTENTS

1. **Introduction to the Second Edition** - 9

2. **What is This Thing Called Harm Reduction in 2025?** – 19

3. **A Little History (of An Often-Overlooked Part) of the Harm Reduction Movement** - 45

Part 1: Policy/Advocates & People Who Use/Used Drugs (PWUD) – 61
    Brian Bourassa - 63
    Joe Clifford - 71
    Laura Guzman - 79
    Tracey Helton - 89
    Kyle Johnston - 97
    Azzy-Mae Ni Mhaille - 109
    Chad Sabora - 117
    Njon Sanders - 129
    Emanuel Sferios - 137
    Chris Steil - 147
    Maia Szalavitz - 153
    Lorie Violette - 163

Part 2: "Boots on the Ground" – Outreach Workers - 171
    Mike Brown - 173
    Michael Kelly - 181
    Erica Poellot - 191
    Tessa Reynolds - 197
    Jess Tilley - 207

Part 3: Treatment – Harm Reduction Counselors/Therapists/ Researchers – 215

  Kenneth Anderson - 217
  Philip Baker (alias) - 225
  Michael Clark - 233
  Susan Collins - 243
  Jennifer Fernandez - 253
  Perri Franskoviak - 259
  Robb Fulghum - 267
  Reid Hester - 273
  Adi Jaffe - 279
  Scott Kellogg - 283
  Gary Langis - 293
  Barry Lessin – 301
  Albie Park - 307
  George Parks - 317
  Jeremy Prillwitz - 331
  Zach Rhoads - 339
  Edith Springer - 345

Part 4: Families & Couples – 349

4. Harm Reduction Psychotherapy with Families & Couples - 351

5. The 3 Worst Words in Addiction Treatment: Codependency, Enabling & Tough Love - 371

  Brenda Zane - 387
  Cathy Taughinbaugh - 391
  Cheryl & Morgan (alias) - 395
  Joan & Doug (alias) - 401
  Jane (alias) - 409
  Susan Ousterman - 418
  Meghann Perry & Sophie Perry-Stewart - 424
  Tori Miller - 442

Index – 446

INTRODUCTION TO THE SECOND EDITION

There are hundreds of paths up the mountain, all leading in the same direction, so it doesn't matter which path you take. The only one wasting time is the one who runs around and around the mountain, telling everyone that their path is wrong.

...Hindu Proverb

I'm finishing the edits of this introduction on August 31, 2024, International Overdose Awareness Day. I've stopped to listen to an event sponsored by the Vilomah Foundation begun by one of the interviewees in this edition[1], Susan Ousterman, who is also sharing, along with three other moms, their individual incredibly painful stories of the loss of their child to overdose. It's heart-wrenching. Listening to how some of these parents were treated by so-called health professionals, as well as some law enforcement, is shocking in its brutality and cruelty. And then when they need a safer space to grieve, they are again turned away. Some don't want to hear about the death of someone from drug use when their child or other loved one died of cancer, or some other illness. This is often because others believe their child's death was due to no fault of their own, both the family's efforts and of course the child's. They are innocent. However, when you lose anyone due to substances, but *especially* a child, many will claim that the parents or partners negligence plays a role somehow. Comments such as, *"If you'd been a better parent, you would've known something was wrong." "Why didn't you stop them from using drugs?" or "How could you possibly not know your partner was drinking so much!"* Some will even say this loved one deserved to overdose, that it's the fault of their own use of drugs. Think about that for a moment—and then ask yourself, "Who are we? Who would be so cruel to a parent or partner or friend or anyone who just lost someone they loved?" The answer to those questions reminds me of this quote from an old comic strip: "We have met the enemy and he is us."[2] Indeed.

When I wrote *Kicking & Screaming* 15 years ago, the world was a very different place in so many way—and so was addiction treatment. Today in the field of addiction we know much more about who is more likely to develop a disorder—and why—though we also have much more to discover. For instance, we have more proof that the brain is flexible, termed *neuroplasticity*[3]. This concept tells us that our environment, the food we eat, even learning can all repair much (most?) of the damage that may have been done through substance use. We now better understand that addiction is at least in great part a learned behavior, which means it can be *unlearned*.[4] We also know more convincingly that substance use disorder is not a chronic, lifelong diagnosis for everyone. Again, the brain's neuroplasticity, or ability to heal and change, shows us that being *recovered* is possible according to Dr. Nora Volkow, head of the National Institute of Drug Abuse or NIDA[5]. These changes and others are significant for treatment options and research but also how we view addiction, which means how we see those who use drugs, including alcohol and tobacco. Today we have a crisis of overdose deaths by various mainly illicit substances and mixing of substances. According to a new RAND study[6], *more than 40 percent of Americans know someone who has died of a drug overdose and about one-third of those individuals say their lives were disrupted by the death.* These are extraordinary numbers and yet we still refuse to do much differently in this country. We are clearly a culture (perhaps a world) in pain. Here in the US, this translates to more than 100,000 deaths from overdose yet too many still demand more punishment, more laws, more crack down on those that use substances—even the friends and low-level drug dealers (like I was) who deal to get their drugs for lower costs—rather than realize that these are the very policies that got us here to begin with: The War on Drugs[7] has been waged for more than 50 years now and has cost us in the US at least *$1 trillion* dollars. Have these efforts led to a reduction of addiction or even drug use? No. We don't need more policies or laws based on anger, and hate, and pain; people who use drugs are often already in pain of all kinds. I sure was. While I may have begun to use substances to escape, to be "cool" and fit into a group, or to "feel better," no one uses substances problematically for 20 years because it's fun[8]. No one.

This also seems a good place to give you the four questions that I asked all interviewees:

- *How did you come to harm reduction?*

- *What's your definition of harm reduction?*

- *What's one thing you really wish others would understand better about harm reduction?*

- *Where would you like to see harm reduction in the future?*

Sometimes the answer to those questions will be brief or more direct. Other times, those I spoke to took time to spin a terrific tale or share some things that they hadn't thought about for a while; often they discussed other people they worked with and befriended due to harm reduction, especially people we have lost—many whom I interviewed for the first edition. This is also part of working in harm reduction and harm reduction psychotherapy.

You may notice that these stories are different lengths, and each has a unique "voice." This is purposeful. I encouraged people to answer my queries in whatever way they chose. I was also determined to interview a variety of people from all over the country and though I could have done another 40 interviews easily, I had to stop due to time and budget. But I have tried my best to represent a bit of who and what harm reduction is: multidimensional, multicultural, and just plain truly remarkable, special people doing a variety of harm reduction work. And you know what? I think we all work together better than we did 15 years ago when folks tended to "stay in their lane" more. Now with social media, we can better connect and learn who each other is, perhaps see what area of harm reduction we want to focus on but then feel free to cross over into other domains too. It's an exciting time to work in harm reduction regardless of the domain! We are definitely making inroads, and we are still underfunded, overworked, and all too often fighting the same battles we did 15 or 50 years ago … and sometimes fighting with each other, sadly. This work is not for wimps!

Another change in this edition is that the interviews have been broken into four sections, three of them representing the three domains of harm reduction (though there's plenty of crossover in these domains): 1) Policy (some of the leaders or management in harm reduction settings); 2) Outreach (the *Boots on the Ground* bad arses who literally save lives every day), and 3) Treatment & Research. That's where I work and where harm reduction psychotherapy and holistic harm reduction psychotherapy (HRT/HHRT) live too. I've also updated a chapter from the first edition titled, *"What is this Thing called Harm Reduction?"*

Finally, there's a section on *Harm Reduction Psychotherapy with Families & Couples.* This is a brand-new chapter and I'm excited to debut this work here for you! You'll find some case discussions, some interviews with a family or couple and a chapter explaining some of the work that I and a few other harm reductionists are doing with families of all kinds. This is a *work in progress* based on the same harm reduction therapy (HRT) described earlier, meaning it is flexible to be as unique a plan as each family or couple deserves and needs. No one-size-fits-all plans here! So many families are still hearing simplistic, unhelpful and non-scientific answers from too many professionals who still believe these three things: 1) that abstinence is the only good outcome because everyone using substances has a drug problem/is addicted; 2) their loved one needs to go into treatment if there's to be any positive change, and 3) they (the friend, family or partner) is part of the problem. None of these statements are always accurate, even about treatment. While some folks do well in traditional treatment environments, many do not. Researchers Susan Collins[9] and Seema Clifasefi at the University of Washington in Seattle have found that engaging clients in developing their own course of treatment and outcome goals—a modality they call *"HaRT"* or *Harm Reduction Treatment*—is one of the best examples of good treatment leading to positive outcomes of substance use/SUD: fewer days of drug use, greater safety when using substances, and healthier habits all around. There are better ways!

I'm being restored to wonder.

...Unknown

I heard this phrase recently and it had an impact on me. I realized that harm reduction for me has been a restoration, a finding of me, my values (people not things), what fills my heart and soul even though it sometimes hurts too. Harm reduction forces me to manage my own anxiety about people's risky behaviors! That's the thing about it that I love and that also scares me: it's unpredictable. It's flexible and different for each person, in each circumstance and for each event. Just like people. Each is a unique piece of the puzzle of their own life. And yet we humans, especially we neurodivergent (ND) folks, crave structure. So how do we have some structure without becoming frozen and not be so flexible we ooze out all over? That's the challenge with harm reduction: there's no one perfect way. It's also why I think it's a challenge for so many, including me still at times. (Yes, I'm still learning.) What I am sure of is that perfection (abstinence especially) is pressure. That's not a good nor a bad thing; it just is. In fact, I hope harm reduction is also about finding ways that that pressure can be helpful.

You will still find stories of folks with lived and living experiences of using harm reduction as well as 12 Step and other support groups to help make positive changes in their relationship to substances and other behaviors. My hope is to give you a greater sense of harm reduction, beyond "Narcan & needles" to quote Tripti Choudry from *A Shot in the Dark* syringe services in Phoenix, AZ. [10] I see harm reduction and especially harm reduction psychotherapy as a holistic approach and a better understanding of how harm reduction can be viewed and successfully used in substance use/SUD as it already is in most domains of healthcare. I hope to show you through these amazing stories and commentary that harm reduction is the ONLY real solution we have to the War on Drugs, especially during this current illicit opiate crisis. I also hope this helps you better consider, understand, and examine all three buckets of harm reduction and begins a continuous conversation about who and what we are as harm reductionists as well as who and what we are not, as that needs constant scrutiny. Can we view substance use and other behaviors through a lens of "safe enough" versus perfection? Are we ready to admit and become pragmatic about it?

Also like the first book, this edition could not have happened without a lot of help from a large group of people. And since this isn't the Academy Awards, there's no music to stop me: first, my co-author, Joe Clifford, a former student who once asked me for some help and then foolishly said, *...and if I can ever help you with something...*. He's the real writer here and helped turn many of the interviews I did into the stories you're reading here. I invite you to check out his novels and especially his autobiography, *Junkie Love*, which is incredibly raw. Rachel Moore, another former teaching assistant who became my editor and helped us make certain that this was readable; to Meghann Perry, another real writer who generously offered her wisdom and assistance at various points in the creation of this book; to longtime pal, Kenneth Anderson, developer of HAMS online support, who did the indexing; to my hedgie pal Down Under, Helen Mentha, another creative who pushed me to keep going; best friends David MacBryde, Kyla Huckerby and Lyn Williams who always believe in me and without whom I don't know that I'd be here; a special thanks to my "sister," Dr. Lisa Moore, who graciously gave us her time to review chapters and helped me organize my thinking about harm reduction a little differently this time around; to my incredibly gifted (and Clio-Award™ winning) son, Jesse Lee Stout, who designed the cover art for both books and who, with my "daughter-in-law" Cristina Acevedo, offered me literal *refuge in the desert* to work more quietly, until they brought my grandgrrl Cairo—*Petunia* to me. It's for her and all other Gen Alphas, that I do this work and why both Joe and I care so deeply about all people who use drugs of all kinds and in all ways; and lastly to every single interviewee here, and all the other incredible people out there doing selfless work in harm reduction that I didn't get to speak to, **THANK YOU.** I'm truly sorry there wasn't more time to get all the stories I wanted and that should be here. We hope you feel that the folks I did interview in each domain represents you well. Please remember, you matter and we see you. Lastly, we thank those of you reading especially those who use drugs—of any kind, in any way. We hope that you find something of value here too because you are why we do this work, and you are so worth it. To quote the late Dan Bigg, cofounder of The Chicago Recovery Alliance (CRA), *All lives are worth saving.* And I would add this to Dan's quote, *All lives are worth saving, **just as they are**.* That's harm reduction.

We truly hope you enjoy this book but even if you don't, we're always open for comments. You can reach me through my website at deedeestoutconsulting.com and Joe at joeclifford.com. We'd love to hear from you. And now, *on with the show!*

Endnotes

1. Susan Ousterman's story can be found in the section on Harm Reduction for Families & Couples

2. Quote from the Pogo comic strip by Walt Kelly.

3. One of the earliest champions of the idea was Adolf Meyer (1866–1950), the prominent chair of psychiatry at Johns Hopkins University from 1910 to 1941. Meyer spearheaded efforts to transform psychiatry into a clinical discipline situated in university hospitals. He exercised unparalleled influence over the specialty's professional and pedagogical standards in the 20th century. As a theoretician, however, he was criticized and even ridiculed for his insistence that the mind–body divide was an erroneous construct that contradicted the principles of biology and the latest neuroscientific evidence. Lamb S. *Neuroplasticity: A Century-old Idea Championed by Adolf Meyer*. CMAJ. 2019 Dec 9;191(49):E1359-E1361. doi: 10.1503/cmaj.191099. PMID: 31818930; PMCID: PMC6901269.

4. See work by the science writer Maia Szalavitz (who's story can be found in the Policy section) and psychologist & neuroscientist Marc Lewis for more on this subject.

5. https://youtu.be/05PH-IY-ELs?si=2K5Ck7VC7uZRZEMW

6. https://www.rand.org/news/press/2024/02/21.html

7. https://www.nbcnews.com/meet-the-press/data-download/costs-war-drugs-continue-soar-rcna92032

8. I also had no intention of hurting others, only myself.

9. Dr. Susan Collins interview can be found here in the section on "Treatment"

10. https://sitdaz.org/

WHAT IS THIS THING CALLED HARM REDUCTION IN 2025?

Safe supply is what we expect in a society. Whether it be the food we eat, the water we drink or the air we breathe. That expectation does not disappear because someone engages in a behavior others find distasteful. Your life has value whether you drink beer or shoot heroin.

.... Professor Daniel Bear, Hunter College, Toronto, Canada

Since I first wrote this chapter more than fifteen years ago, Harm Reduction (HR) has become something we can actually discuss publicly and nationally—and that's one big positive change! Now we'd like folks to better understand that HR is much more than medications or clean needles; however, these are the parts of HR the media focus on due to the illicit opiate crisis. That's a good thing. But it's not enough. One harm reductionist I interviewed called this part of HR, "the stuff of HR": syringe services programs or SSPs (formerly needle exchange programs): Narcan, drug testing strips, medications, and more. And all of this "stuff" is absolutely crucial to keeping many drug users alive and healthier. Yet, harm reduction has even more to offer than supplies. I have come to see HR in three distinct, often overlapping domains, or "buckets": in no particular order, 1) Policy, 2) Outreach, and 3) Treatment.

Yes, harm reduction (HR) includes treatment! I was disappointed recently to hear a self-professed harm reductionist on a podcast state, "...[t]here is no harm reduction treatment."[1] Ouch. And incorrect. The late G. Alan Marlatt, PhD[2], who pioneered US research and treatment on harm reduction (and more) and who wrote the seminal book, *Harm Reduction*[3] in 1998, discusses HR in many areas including *treatment*: behavioral therapies, moderation in alcohol use, HIV risk reduction in drug users, integrating HR with psychotherapy, methadone maintenance, and more. His book was the first time Harm Reduction had been discussed in the US academically, and it spawned two (2) other important books on HR psychotherapy or *treatment*: first, in 2000, Patt Denning, PhD, a psychologist in San Francisco, CA, wrote *Practicing Harm Reduction Psychotherapy* (with a second edition in 2012 co-authored by Jeannie Little, LCSW, who co-founded the Harm Reduction Therapy Center with Dr. Denning in SF); and then in 2002, Andrew Tatarsky, PhD, another psychologist, this time in New York City, penned *Harm Reduction Psychotherapy*. These two books were the foundation most of us Next Gen harm reduction psychotherapists were schooled on (in addition to numerous trainings from one or both of these and other HR Oldtimers.[4]) And, of course, Dr. Marlatt mentored most of us as well.

I also feel that we need to discuss definitions of harm reduction since we are seeing many organizations state they are "doing/providing harm reduction services" but mainly they are "allowing" clients to continue or sometimes begin a course of their various medications, primarily for Opiate Use Disorder (OUD). It's clear to most of us that these organizations are not truly practicing harm reduction as a milieu culture but are providing harm reduction-informed services; in other words, they have none of the real social justice/anti-War on Drugs culture of HR but rather are offering good medical practices, by providing (or "allowing") the use of various medications.

So, let's take these parts of HR separately as I believe they each play an important role in the definition of HR but also how we view and practice harm reduction and harm reduction psychotherapies today.

Harm Reduction in Policy

The first definition of Harm Reduction is from Harm Reduction International[5]:

Harm reduction refers to policies, programs and practices that aim to minimize the negative health, social and legal impacts associated with drug use, drug policies and drug laws.

Harm reduction is grounded in justice and human rights. It focuses on positive change and on working with people without judgement, coercion, discrimination, or requiring that people stop using drugs as a precondition of support.

Similarly, the definition from the National Harm Reduction Coalition[6] states,

Harm reduction is a set of practical strategies and ideas aimed at reducing negative consequences associated with drug use. Harm Reduction is also a movement for social justice built on a belief in, and respect for, the rights of people who use drugs.

Harm reduction incorporates a spectrum of strategies that in-

cludes safer use, managed use, abstinence, meeting people who use drugs "where they're at," and addressing conditions of use along with the use itself. Because harm reduction demands that interventions and policies designed to serve people who use drugs reflect specific individual and community needs, there is no universal definition of or formula for implementing harm reduction.

National Harm Reduction Coalition works for the Harm Reduction movement built on a belief in and respect for the rights of people who use drugs. Our strategies include building leadership among people who use drugs and supporting communities in reducing the negative consequences associated with drug use. (https://harmreduction.org/movement/)

Finally, here's the definition from the Drug Policy Alliance (DPA)[7]:

Harm reduction is a set of ideas and interventions that seek to reduce the harms associated with both drug use and punitive drug policies. For example, using naloxone reverses an opioid overdose. Not sharing needles reduces the risk of contracting infectious diseases. At Drug Policy Alliance, we advocate to expand harm reduction services across the United States.

Looking at these three definitions, I believe it suddenly becomes clear why harm reduction psychotherapy or treatment has been left out of most conversations about harm reduction as only one organization mentions interventions (which in this case does not mean the kind that is a precursor to treatment-by-surprise. Interventions in healthcare refers to any type of treatment or strategy, such as counseling or medical exams). And the interventions mentioned don't seem to include counseling or therapy.

A few things become apparent with these definitions: 1) harm reduction is a culture, a movement of individuals and organizations that believe in respecting the autonomy of all, which includes the concept of social justice; 2) it's *a way of being with people* (thank you Carl Rogers[8]); and 3) it can—and does—mean different factions of harm reduction may have different focal points depending on the environment and organization in which they're working. Harm reduction can mean everything from abstinence, sober-curious, moderation, abstinence sampling[9], or using some substances and not others—sometimes called *Cali Sober*—and others. It also means we don't *advocate* for abstinence (while we might suggest it for *some* people who use drugs, it's always *their* decision). Again, this does *not* mean that we don't believe in abstinence. It simply means that we don't believe in forcing it on people any more than we believe people should be forced to take medications or to eat more healthily, even though both could be really good for them. Many of us working with people who have problematic relationships with drugs will admit that it would likely be helpful for many of them to stop the substances they're using, but it's not our decision to make. And we definitely believe that all people, even those who use substances problematically or chaotically, have the right to refuse treatment as well as the right to receive care that fits them. Since one of the basic ingredients in HRT is self-determination, we don't *force* people into things, but we sure can—and do have—meaningful, deep conversations to help folks make better-informed decisions of their own. In fact, that's literally our job.

I often see clients when they are under the influence of substances, which was a huge "no-no" when I was trained as an alcohol and other drugs (AOD) counselor (most therapists and counselors still refuse to see a client who's under the influence). I'm surprised when clients are willing to see me when they're intoxicated for a few reasons but first, how come they do this? Here are some answers to that question based on actual statements from clients: 1) allowing me to see them in this state can be quite revealing and insightful—regardless of what most of us have been taught, 2) it's a sign of trust in me, which I appreciate, and 3) counseling sessions to examine possibly changing entrenched behaviors can be stressful and some clients need to imbibe in order to help with that discomfort—until they learn other ways to cope, if possible. But in this moment they're in my office, real or virtual, and I have learned to appreciate that simple fact. As Steve Rollnick[10] has taught me, "If someone's in your office, they're motivated for something!" I've also learned to be constantly curious and respectful to those who come under the influence and to see this behavior as motivation to contemplate a change or willingness to examine what that might be like.

There are also **8 Principles of Harm Reduction**[11] that should be included at this point to perhaps best illustrate what we mean by individuals and organizations being truly harm reduction-informed:

Accepts, for better or worse, that licit and illicit drug use is part of our world and chooses to work to minimize its harmful effects rather than simply ignore or condemn them

Understands drug use as a complex, multi-faceted phenomenon that encompasses a continuum of behaviors from severe use to total abstinence, and acknowledges that some ways of using drugs are clearly safer than others

Establishes quality of individual and community life and well-being—not necessarily cessation of all drug use—as the criteria for successful interventions and policies

Calls for the non-judgmental, non-coercive provision of services and resources to people who use drugs and the communities in which they live in order to assist them in reducing attendant harm

Ensures that people who use drugs and those with a history of drug use routinely have a real voice in the creation of programs and policies designed to serve them

Affirms people who use drugs (PWUD) themselves as the primary agents of reducing the harms of their drug use and seeks to empower PWUD to share information and support each other in strategies [that] meet their actual conditions of use

Recognizes that the realities of poverty, class, racism, social isolation, past trauma, sex-based discrimination, and other social inequalities affect both people's vulnerability to and capacity for effectively dealing with drug-related harm

Does not attempt to minimize or ignore the real and tragic harm and danger that can be associated with illicit drug use

These are all excellent conceptualizations of harm reduction. However the ones I use and reference most often are the "6 *Basic Principles of Harm Reduction for Healthcare Settings*[12]" simply because these are the usual settings in which I am providing training in various subjects on or related to harm reduction. These are:

Humanism: all people are deserving of compassionate healthcare; humans behave for reasons & providers need to understand those reasons

Pragmatism: no one is perfect in their health behavior; health behaviors are influenced by social determinants such as environment

Individualism: all humans have strengths and needs; folks come with a spectrum of harms, motivation, & willingness so we need interventions appropriate to each point on that spectrum

Autonomy: providers can make suggestions [or] give advice with permission but ultimately decisions are up to the individual based on their situation, environment, beliefs, and priorities

Incrementalism: any positive change is change; change can take years & many attempts so providers need to be prepared

Accountability without Termination: people are responsible for their own behaviors & decisions; clients aren't "fired" for not reaching their goals; people have the right to make unhealthy decisions for themselves & providers can empathetically still help them to understand that those decisions may have serious outcomes that are their own. Even steps back aren't punished but rather are compassionately understood and expected[13]

There has been and still is a lot of misunderstanding about harm reduction, along with many distracting and wrong-headed myths concerning its principles and practice, which have led directly to much of the controversy surrounding it. Sometimes people have simply misinterpreted or inaccurately stated the goals or ethics of the agencies, municipalities, or people implementing different aspects of harm reduction. Often, however, these misunderstandings have led to core challenges of harm reduction policies by those who advocate for abstinence-only treatment for any drug use, addiction/SUD or not.

Since transparency is a major point of harm reduction policy, let me shed a little sunshine on some of these controversies and misinterpretations while developing a working definition of harm reduction as I go along.

Myth #1: Harm reduction is the opposite of abstinence.

Abstinence is and always has been one of the possible outcomes of harm reduction treatment. Abstinence is found on the continuum of drug use used in harm reduction theory and practice[14], although one could accurately say it's on one end of a continuum and is one possibility in a menu of outcome options a client might choose. In fact, it could be argued that harm reduction puts abstinence in perspective and sees how it may not be the right fit for everyone, which we know is accurate[15]. You might look at it this way: *abstinence from anything equals perfection*. As we are human and, therefore, by definition imperfect, the much-observed inability to be perfectly abstinent (the tendency to relapse or slip) often leads us to feeling shameful when we inevitably behave as a human being does, i.e., we *make a mistake*. And, ironically, the shame we feel as a result of not being able to maintain anything like "perfect adherence"[16] to this desired outcome of abstinence often leads us right back to the behavior we're trying to avoid or stop. This is what the late author and researcher G. Alan Marlatt called the *abstinence violation effect*, or AVE, in his book on *Relapse Prevention*[17].

Back in early AA, this idea of perfection was a topic that was often discussed. In fact, this concern led the early groups to embrace those who "slipped" or "lapsed"—drank alcohol again—to help reduce the shame those members often felt, as everyone recognized no one among them was perfect. Coming to the aid of a "lapsed" member was also thought to help other members avoid the pitfalls that had led to that member's "slip"; it was seen as a learning opportunity for all members. This was when the AA slogan "progress not perfection" started to be heard.

Therefore, our thoughts on harm reduction begins with the premise that there is a menu of options, including abstinence, available to PWUD seeking help or in treatment, and only they alone can ultimately make the choice to abstain or to moderate, or be Cali-sober, or something else including to continue their behavior "as is." Harm reduction, along with AA as described above, clearly recognizes in its notion of choice that no one is perfect and attempts to build in a process towards health or wellness (recovery) that is personal, appropriate to the individual, and seeks to avoid shaming PWUD for their inability to be perfect. In other words, we see human beings as human—as did AA! Harm reduction also believes that people make their own choices best after getting accurate and impartial information on all the possible options available to them, including the pros and cons of each, and various supports available. With this, people will have what they need to make better, more informed decisions.

Myth #2: Clinicians should be in charge of treatment, not clients.

Typically, we think of treatment as a group of professionals or an agency making decisions for clients based on the belief that 1) clients can't make healthy decisions for themselves (*"your best thinking got you here"*) and 2) we're the experts, so we logically know how best to treat this (these) condition(s). But are these beliefs true? We harm reductionists would say "not necessarily." We would certainly agree that there are occasions when folks might need additional help in their decision-making processes, and we'd even agree that occasionally someone might be so ill that a single decision could need to be made for them *in the moment*. We would, however, strongly disagree with those who say we must make *all* decisions for *all* drug users as long as they're using. Why do we disagree? Well, for one, because we *do* believe that their best thinking got them "here"—to us or some other type of help for those who want to examine their relationship to a drug! And 2) because we also know that most drug users don't have and never will have a problem with their drug use.

We also know that different drugs interact with each individual user differently. Therefore, we must form professional opinions and policies based on the individual in front of us, on their behavior and desires, and their support networks, and not on the particular drug they are using. Good treatment helps PWUD to examine their relationship to this drug (or drugs) in its entirety: the good, the bad, and the ugly; warts and all. We do this through asking about and listening to the individual's history, their physiology, the context of their use, the particular drug and how it's being used, plus their desired outcome or goals of treatment. In other words, all decisions regarding treatment options must be made by PWUD. So a good treatment might say, "Since you have a family who cares, work you enjoy, and a desire to reduce your use of alcohol, what do *you* think would be helpful to help you continue to moderate?" And if I as a professional felt that I wanted to share my thoughts with this client, I would merely ask to do so. In other words, "I wonder if I could share some of my ideas for treatment possibilities that I think could help you make an even more informed decision?" Most people are more than happy to hear our opinions; they simply want to be respected for having their own as well. Therefore, to extend our developing thoughts on harm reduction and to counter Myth #2, we might say that respecting the opinions, choices, and goals—including the goal to be abstinent or not—of the individual seeking help is *always* the most important aspect of harm reduction therapy, theory, and practice.

Myth #3: Harm reduction is just giving people permission to use drugs/engage in bad behavior.

OK, this is the Big One. And the smart-aleck response from me is this: personally, never *ever* in 20 years of using various drugs did I ever ask *anybody* for permission to use *anything*, so this statement is completely ridiculous. And that's the truth. Whenever I've asked other former or current users if they ever asked permission from someone before they used a drug of any kind, I've never received an affirmative response. But seriously, let's discuss this issue a bit further as I do think it's an important one.

This idea of "giving permission" implies first off that I somehow *can* give permission to another person. But as a fellow human being, I can neither give nor take permission from another not under my legal care, especially around the issue of using a substance or other risky behaviors. First of all, it's simply not possible: how would I do such a thing? I might believe that I have such power but, in reality, that is hubris. Now what I might have over someone is *leverage*, which is different. The difference is this: power implies that I, through my own desires, can make you do something. For example, let's say I'm taller and stronger than you so I can force you to be polite to me. *Leverage* means I can persuade, threaten, or cajole you into doing something, such as making a change. Now usually this is true because I can make good on a threat to something/against

30

someone you want or care for. I can blackmail you to do something for instance. Very different. Furthermore, in the context of the criminal legal system, I can send people to jail, or back to jail, or take them away from their families, but how can I be sure that they will show up to jail as opposed to running off to another country? Or in drug treatment, how can I be sure someone *never* uses alcohol or other drugs again? I can't be with them all the time, and drug tests only tell me what someone *might* have done (past tense) not what they're doing right now, so that's not really a helpful measurement in this case (and drug tests aren't infallible). Leverage goes only so far, even in a coercive system such as the criminal legal system.

So this means that there must be some buy-in from PWUD, some agreement on their part in order for them to really get help, right? Harm reduction approaches have been shown to increase one's motivation toward change (including, in many cases, towards abstinence), often even more than traditional treatment approaches, in part through the addition of that personal buy in[18]. Isn't that remarkable? And you know, when left with the choice in treatment or therapy to be abstinent or moderate in their drinking, many people wind up deciding to be abstinent—on their own, based on their own examination of their behavior. Colleagues and I have compared notes, and we find that clients often say that abstinence is just easier than trying to moderate and track drinks, or that it isn't nearly as much fun if you can't get drunk (yes, responsible drinking means not getting drunk regularly). In general, we see that people naturally want to be healthier; it's just that we humans are so darned hard-wired to resist change that we often will do anything to avoid it—sometimes even when we know it's best for us. And by the way, that's not denying the need for change—or being *in denial*—that's just being human!

31

So, in shattering Myth #3, we include in our growing thoughts on harm reduction the fact that, far from giving people permission to use, harm reduction and harm reduction psychotherapy helps uncover the internal motivations in people and supports their natural instinct towards healthier, and maybe even abstinent, behavior. This includes exploring the motivations of people's behavior through posing some challenging questions and using artful reflections and more to help people come to terms with the discrepancies in their goals, values, and behaviors—not in a "get in your face" way but in an honest way: how is (are) your current behavior(s) helping or hindering you from getting the goals you want in life? What/how would you like to change your relationship to substances/behaviors. If you decide to make a change at all?

Myth #4: You can't mix harm reduction and abstinence goals in treatment/harm reduction means anything goes.

I thought I would combine these last two as they are intricately related. First of all, I've often heard that we can't mix goals in treatment: clients who want to abstain will be triggered by those who do not wish to or who are under-the-influence in the milieu. I've also heard, consistently, that there are liability issues for agencies, which is why they don't allow anyone who is under the influence of drugs to be on the premises, client or not.

Realistically, if you walk into almost any 12 Step meeting, and possibly other mutual aid groups, at any time, you're likely to sit next to someone who is under the influence of some drug, often alcohol. And, amazingly, no one tells them to leave, and no one gets upset that they're being "triggered," in spite of the abstinence-only message many receive in 12 Step meetings. In fact, members are often the kindest to those who come to meetings under the influence (perhaps we're reminded of where we came from—and where we could be again?). I have heard the secretary of a meeting kindly suggest—*not insist*—that any persons under the influence might just want to listen today instead of speaking ("sharing" it's called) but, mostly, that person would simply be invited to "Keep Coming Back!"[19]

As for the oft-repeated statement that harm reduction means "anything goes," I offer the following: Harm reduction psychotherapy is a complicated combination of accurate education, different therapeutic models, often medications, skill-building, nutritional and somatic supports, therapeutic aid for family and concerned others, and much more. It is the most comprehensive treatment I know. Again, this long-held myth that harm reduction simply means the client does whatever they want, with no consequence, is silly at best and a lie at worst. No harm reductionist would want someone to drive a car under the influence of a drug that could impair their ability to safely navigate a road. But we might advocate for treatment over jail time. Or better yet, why don't we install breathalyzers everywhere alcohol is served as well as in vehicles? Wouldn't prevention be far better than punishment after the fact? We agree that people must be held responsible for their actions; we also want to do our best to understand why someone behaved as they did and offer compassion rather than judgment. In fact, that is the very point: we harm reductionists don't care as much about what or how someone uses a drug as we care about **how you behave under its influence**. So, far from being an "anything goes" policy or treatment approach, harm reduction is the *gold-standard* for holding people responsible; we simply do this with deep compassion and less judgment. So, what does harm reduction treatment look like in an agency setting? Good question!

Since harm reduction is all about *reducing* harm, not increasing it, we agree that facilities, agencies, workers and policy makers need guidelines—just not as many as they may think they need. Guidelines—safety tenets, rules, agreements, whatever you may call them—aren't reasons for unilateral prohibitions such as discharging clients who use drugs or engage in other behaviors that led them to treatment in the first place. Let's say that again: we should not discharge clients *for exhibiting the very behavior(s) for which they are in treatment!* Substance-use disorder is a mental health condition amongst other domains; it's found in the DSM5-TR, the guidebook for mental health conditions including substance-use disorders. So how has it happened that substance-use disorders get viewed differently from other disorders or medical conditions? How is it that treatment for this illness does not allow people to show any visible *signs* of that disorder (using drugs, resisting treatment options, ambivalence about making changes, acting out their trauma responses, etc.), especially in light of the fact that this *is why they chose to* seek *help?* Think about it: if you were having heart problems and you came to the emergency department in the midst of a heart attack, would someone suggest that you needed to "just stop having heart attacks first" or "come back when you're really ready to stop having heart attacks and take this seriously," which might include having to give up your job, your home, your family and friends, and your main coping mechanism (the substance use/other risky behavior) in order to just *get help?* Furthermore, once a person *does* decide to enter drug treatment of some kind to examine and perhaps change their relationship to a substance(s), if their symptoms return, why are *they* blamed most often instead of looking at the *treatment* as possibly ineffective for that person? Providers are guilty of blaming and/or punishing "patients/clients" by discharging them, withholding treatments, or labeling them as "resistant," "antisocial/borderline," "being in denial," and more. We providers rarely admit it could be *our* treatment that has failed. (I suggested this once and was told we couldn't do that, i.e., admit to possible failure of treatment, because we'd be open to a lawsuit). And, more importantly, how is it that *our* punitive behavior is not completely unethical?

So, to integrate these concepts into our thoughts on harm reduction, we can see that, far from a philosophy of "anything goes," harm reduction is dedicated to treating a PWUD regardless of where on the spectrum of drug use (or change) that person is, and it does not withhold treatment or care based on some fixed and predetermined judgment having *nothing* to do with the unique circumstances of that individual.

The final thought on harm reduction treatment here involves an ethical and compassionate acceptance of the whole person, combined with a collaborative approach, whose goal is to help individuals improve their lives—to get closer to their goals in ways that make sense to *them* and are possible within *that* person's abilities and resources—regardless of whether they use a substance or engage in other risky behaviors ... *one baby step at a time.* Change is a slow and unsteady process most of the time and definitely for those of us with a challenging relationship to a drug/behavior we've used for some time. As Alan Marlatt once said to me, "We don't budget enough for change." Boy, was he right!

One of the main skills I've had to learn in practicing HRT or any modality with PWUD and other risky behaviors is to manage my own anxiety—and I *do* have anxiety about people's behaviors sometimes because I'm human! This can mean I need to seek consultation with a colleague or friend, perhaps someone not in the field (they often provide me with a unique perspective). Perhaps I need to do some added research about the behavior or drug that's being used. Perhaps I need to go for a walk, do a breathing exercise, or another somatic therapy. Perhaps I need to apologize to my client, admit that the anxiety is *my* issue and that it's temporarily clouded my perspective. Yes, I've had to do that on occasion (even recently) and asked to start over with that client, promising to listen more and deal with my anxiety on my time, not theirs. This dis-*ease*, as the late John Bradshaw[20] would call addiction, is real with all risky behaviors, and because our culture fails to help folks cope with, or even recognize, dis-*ease* or anxiety in a healthier way, we too often wind up transferring our anxiety into trying to force people to make changes in ways that *we* want—that we are convinced will alleviate *our* anxiety—and not necessarily the ones that they want. (If you need proof, I suggest revisiting Pixar's *Inside Out* films.)

Ultimately, our cultural conceptualization of harm reduction and the myths surrounding it appear to come down to beliefs more often than science. Even members of my own profession often act as if these myths or mistaken beliefs about harm re-duction are true rather than seeking out accurate information. In 12 Step language, I could say we have been sorely lacking in "honesty, open mindedness and willingness[21]" to see harm reduction for what it really is: *pragmatic strategies for manag-ing high-risk behaviors,* to quote the subtitle of the late G. Alan Marlatt's book, *Harm Reduction*[22]. And, bottom line, the health and lives of people with addictions/SUD is far too important to continue acting out these differences amongst ourselves or with PWUD, our clients.

Interestingly, it seems that government health organizations are redefining recovery these days, using more HR-informed language. The Substance Abuse and Mental Health Services Administration (SAMHSA) redefined recovery a few years ago. Here is their current definition: *[A] process of change that involves: Improving health and wellness, [l]iving a self-directed life, and [s]triving to reach one's full potential.*[23] In 2022, the National Institute on Alcohol Abuse and Alcoholism (NIAAA) also offered a new definition of recovery, this one specific to Alcohol Use Disorder, or AUD, since that's their only scope of research:

Recovery is a process through which an individual pursues both remission from alcohol use disorder (AUD) and cessation from heavy drinking.[24](added emphasis mine). They go on to say that a state of being "recovered" is also possible: *An individual may be considered "recovered" if both remission from AUD and cessation from heavy drinking are achieved and maintained over time. For those experiencing alcohol-related functional impairment and other adverse consequences, recovery is often marked by the fulfillment of basic needs, enhancements in social support and spirituality, and improvements in physical and mental health, quality of life, and other dimensions of well-being*[25].

Well, so much for the lifetime, chronic, progressive diseased state of addiction/SUD we here in the States have promoted for decades!

One final addition in this conversation about the disease concept of addiction/SUD: while it's becoming more and more accepted that SUDs are not a disease, certainly not a brain disease, perhaps it becomes one for some. After a fascinating training on the subject many years ago with a professor in pharmacology from the University of Texas at Austin, I had one of my last conversations with Dr. Alan Marlatt. I explained to him that this professor and researcher suggested that maybe for a very few, some 1 – 3% and usually with a family history of addiction who can't seem to stop unless confined, they develop this disease state. I asked Alan what he thought about this idea, and he said he thought it was possible. It made sense to me then and does so even more today since we now view substance use and disorders on a spectrum. This is also what I love—and miss—about Alan so much: he never acted like he knew it all even though he was one of the world's expert researchers and professors on addiction. Rest in Power, my friend and mentor.

Here, I'd also like to add something from AA called the Responsibility Statement that I shared recently with my "sister," Professor Lisa Moore, PhD (whose story is in the first edition) who had never heard this but thought, like me, that it applies in harm reduction work as well: I am responsible.[26] When anyone, anywhere, reaches out for help, I want the hand of AA always to be there. And for that I am responsible. Perhaps this is something we harm reductionists can take from AA—and here's why I say that: I have some concerns about us and the harm reduction movement, and who we may be becoming now. Where is our neutrality, our seeing others as our siblings who all deserve our grace and care? Do we extend that grace to those who are not in our harm reduction communities, or in other communities with which we have disagreement? Have we adopted the robes of the system of oppression (that we've all lived in forever)? Have we become the oppressors? We see this happen in historical movements of all kinds. Why should we be any different? And if that's the case, what do we do about it? How do we stop trying to create safe spaces and accept that the best we can ever do is to create safer spaces, for us and for others?

We see fighting within harm reduction communities exacerbating arguments over funding and, worse, questioning who belongs in our movement and who doesn't, who can speak at conferences (and at which ones), and more. Here are some thoughts I have had on this, which are by no means perfect or right or the only ones we should consider. I simply want to encourage all of us to continue to explore these itchy ideas and be honest, open-minded, and willing to change our individual and collective minds. With these three concepts, we might be able to see harm reduction in all its forms. After all, harm reduction is mutual support just like 12 Step. Supporting one another is a core value along with passing on what we're given. Professor Moore wonders whether we'd be better off viewing harm reduction as a group of communities, contiguous, rather than one humungous, continuous community, as well as asking, "How do we give each other more grace?" Perhaps we need to view more mutual support groups this way as well? What we have in common is core to us all: we are the folks who love and desire to support all people who use drugs (PWUD) of all kinds, right?

So, where does this leave us? I'd argue at the beginning of change. Harm reduction and 12 Step and other mutual support groups offer assistance to PWUD and other marginalized and often vilified people. Many of us have fought for a place to belong, just like the folks we serve. As I write this in late 2024, harm reduction has gone mainstream in many places (New York City; New Jersey; Minnesota, et al., and at the same time, is once again being blamed for increased drug use, homelessness, and crime in others (sadly, San Francisco, CA). Is this finally the moment for all of us—harm reductionists and all mutual aid groups—to come together, to seek understanding and greater partnership (as I argued for back in 2009 in the first edition)? We have so much in common! Yes, I realize that the application of each is complicated and different from each other, and not everyone will seek cooperation. And that's okay. But what if we focused more on our mutually held values than our differences (another value in 12 Step, btw)? Could that cooperation lead to a new focus and help us develop ways to combat the ongoing and horrendously damaging War on Drugs? What do we have to lose?

To finish this revised section, I would like to make some suggested guidelines for us harm reductionists and allies toward a mutually beneficial end to the War on Drugs, as well as on PWUD, to help us gain traction toward seeing more HR/HRT in treatment milieus:

1) There are no harm reduction police so please stop cancelling and bullying each other. This means we need more discourse, more conversation, and not necessarily more social media posts because it's virtually impossible to truly converse on social media. We can begin to have talks, we can organize panels and workshops on the forum, but having deep difficult conversations, which involves nuance and intimacy (among others), is simply too problematic.

2) Let's give everyone the benefit of the doubt first. Before you think the worst of someone, perhaps take a moment to think the best instead.

3) HR is more than "Narcan and needles!"[27] Please stop calling MAT harm reduction. It's not. It's good medicine and it's important. It's just not harm reduction. This has been a way for too many providers to slip into the false "we provide harm reduction services" narrative and the media's reduction of harm reduction to "Narcan and needles"[28]. Harm reduction is a group

of strategies, services, and skills but it is always rooted in social justice. So, if your treatment program provides medication for various medical conditions, like MOUD meds, feel free to state that in bold letters! Just please don't say you're "doing HR" unless you're also willing to embrace the social component. You may freely use the phrase I found at a headshop in Seattle back at my first HR conference, where it was printed on buttons that I still hand out everywhere: Another conscientious objector to the War on Drugs.[29]

4) Expand your knowledge and your network. Include us harm reduction OGs, newbies, those with lived and living experience, as well as those without experience but who are willing to learn about harm reduction/HRT. Take classes, workshops, including ones outside our specific field (I highly suggest Loretta Ross[30]' work on calling people in v out but there are many worthwhile others out there at reasonable cost). Study other areas of health or public policy or modalities of health as you're interested and able. Let's all jump into the deep end of our collective harm reduction pool and help each other stay afloat. Because that's what harm reduction is all about: helping others.

The last word in this revised section on harm reduction thoughts, principles, and myths will be coming from another couple of Harm Reduction Oldtimers from my first edition, and one in which I believe we can all agree: "Recovery (and harm reduction) is any positive change," and we all want to help people make positive changes in their lives—as long as they are changes that they want to make, when they are ready to make them (though we can gently encourage someone to get thirsty for change!), and in a way that makes sense/is most probable to happen for them. What I love most about the simple phrase of "any positive change" is that it was first spoken, not by our late harm reduction leader and my friend, the late Dan Bigg (Founder, CRA, Chicago Recovery Alliance) as I had once thought, but rather by a 12 Step loving, regular meeting-attending, heroin-using gentle man named John Szyler, aka "Division Street." John died of an overdose in May 1996 but not before giving us these few extraordinary words: Recovery is any positive change. What better way to describe harm reduction too! I hope his legacy will not be simply as a drug user, but rather as a visionary who happened to use drugs sometimes, like we all do (I had my caffeine and pain meds this morning. How about you?); someone who helped us come together as peers, professionals and folks who care deeply about our fellow humans who are also drug users—who love PWUD. I also think of John as someone who aided us in our desire to stop letting politics—and which mutual-aid camp we're in—interfere with what our hearts all know is true: that all lives are indeed worth saving, and that any positive change is the best way to help make that happen. Lastly, perhaps this conversation, rather than controversy and debate, could continue if we were to trust in this quote from Johann Wolfgang von Goethe , the late German writer and philosopher, one that I ran across in graduate school: *Treat people as if they are what they can be, and you help them to become who they're capable of being.* And that is still one of my favorite quotes to define "harm reduction."

Endnotes

1. As I have no wish to publicly call out this person, their name and that of the podcast will remain anonymous.

2. Dr. Marlatt was an award-winning Canadian American author and Professor of Psychology as well as the longtime Director of the Addictive Behaviors Research Center at the University of Washington, Seattle until his death in 2011.

3. Marlatt, G. Alan, Editor. (1998). *Harm Reduction: Pragmatic Strategies for Managing High-Risk Behaviors.* The Guilford Press, NY/London.

4. More on the stories of these harm reduction pioneers, including Jeannie Little, LCSW, co-founder with Dr. Denning of the Harm Reduction Therapy Center in San Francsico, can be found in the first edition of *Coming to Harm Reduction Kicking & Screaming* in the section on "Harm Reduction Oldtimers."

5. https://hri.global/what-is-harm-reduction/. Accessed 9.3.24.

6. https://harmreduction.org/wp-content/uploads/2022/12/NHRC-PDF-Principles_Of_Harm_Reduction.pdf. Accessed 9.3.24

7. https://drugpolicy.org/harmreduction/. Accessed 9.3.24.

8. https://en.wikipedia.org/wiki/Carl_Rogers

9. https://www.igntd.com/the-blog/abstinence-sampling. Accessed 9.7.2024.

10. Co-author of Motivational Interviewing. More on his work can be found here: https://www.stephenrollnick.com/

11. https://harmreduction.org/about-us/principles-of-harm-reduction/

12. Hawk M, Coulter RWS, Egan JE, Fisk S, Reuel Friedman M, Tula M, Kinsky S. Harm reduction principles for healthcare settings. Harm Reduct J. 2017 Oct 24;14(1):70. doi: 10.1186/s12954-017-0196-4. PMID: 29065896; PMCID: PMC5655864.

13. https://harmreductionjournal.biomedcentral.com/articles/10.1186/s12954-017-0196-4/tables/1

14. See "The Continuum of Alcohol and other Drug Use" chart by Jeannie Little, Director, Harm Reduction Therapy Center, in the Appendix.

15. https://www.recoveryanswers.org/research-post/in-recovery-non-abstinent-approaches-common-through-abstinence-associated-better-quality-life/

16. From Alcoholics Anonymous, 4th Edition, (2008) AAWS. Online version. p. 60.

17. Marlatt, G.A. & Gordon, J.M. *Relapse Prevention*. (1985). The Guilford Press. NY/London.

18. See Miller & Rollnick, Motivational Interviewing 4th Edition (2023) for more.

19. This compassion is not shown in all 12 Step meetings, however. Sadly, some members indeed do shame folks who have returned to their old behavior. This is not supported by Central Office or literature, but members may behave differently as there is no 12 Step "police" or monitors. Gratefully in this case, each meeting can be run as the group decides.

20. See https://en.wikipedia.org/wiki/John_Bradshaw_(author) for more.

21. https://www.aa.org/sites/default/files/2021-11/en_bigbook_appendiceii.pdf

22. Marlatt, G. A. (1998) Harm Reduction. The Guilford Press. NY, NY.

23. https://www.samhsa.gov/sites/default/files/samhsa-recovery-5-6-14.pdf

24. https://www.niaaa.nih.gov/research/niaaa-recovery-from-alcohol-use-disorder/definitions

25. Ibid.

26. For more on this Statement, see https://www.aacle.org/history-behind-aas-responsibility-statement/

27. Personal communication with Tripti Choudry, HR outreach worker, clinician and colleague. November 2024.

28. Ibid.

29. Many orgs are willing to provide Naloxone, buprenorphine, Narcan which are all vital supplies of HR outreach but they don't/won't use HRT or embed the principles & policies of HR in their milieu or treatment. This is what actually determines whether an org or individual is practicing HR or are possibly "HR-informed" or simply providing good medical treatment.

30. https://www.youtube.com/watch?v=xw_720iQDss. Here's her TEDTalk from 2022 on the subject

A LITTLE HISTORY (OF AN OFTEN-OVERLOOKED PART) OF THE HARM REDUCTION MOVEMENT

Whoever saves a single life is considered by scripture to have saved the whole world.

...Jewish saying from the Talmud

Note: Since we often discuss the history of harm reduction through the lens of academia and white culture, I thought it would be more interesting here to view it through others' lenses. What follows is terribly incomplete and brief, but I hope it gives you a taste of some of the other important contributions of BIPOC, 2SLGBTQIA and other overlooked communities to the origins of HR.

In Midland, MI, in the early 1970s, I was part of a small group of teens being trained in how to handle "bad trips" by local psychologist Dr. Don Crowder (who was also my doctor). Dr. Crowder wanted to open a safe space for teens who were experimenting with drugs—mainly hallucinogens (plus alcohol of course)—as well as train a few teens to help their friends. Teens were using such large amounts that they were at risk for reoccurring, lifelong problems in this mainly white, upper middle-class to high socio-economic town, (please know that my hometown was, and is, the international headquarters for Dow Chemical—Saran Wrap, Ziplock bags, and napalm bombs. Go Dow!). Dr. Crowder understood these well-off kids had the resources, i.e., time and money, to be using drugs far more often and in greater amounts than those not in those wealthy circles. (My dad was one of the few in town who *didn't* work for Dow). When the City Council heard what Dr. Crowder had planned, they quickly shut him down, saying, "We don't have a drug problem in Midland, Michigan!" Right. No one wanted to listen to his prescient pleading. Sadly, this training to reduce the potential harm to teens never got beyond that initial effort, but it left an impression on me even though I had been using drugs since age twelve. It took me nearly twenty years more to realize that this was early harm reduction work.

Midland was a town of about thirty thousand in those days, and not a great example of harm reduction overall (as you just read). It was also mainly white. I can recall precisely when the first two Black families moved in. They worked for Dow. The son of one family beat me out for Class President at Northeast Junior High; the other became members of our church, Midland United Church of Christ, where I taught their sons Sunday School. Slowly it made me wonder if other communities, especially where drug use was even more prevalent, were able to hear those early messages of reducing harm for their residents engaged in risky behaviors and using illicit substances? What was happening in the big cities, which were now predominately populated by People of Color and others marginalized? Surely they would heed these messages of help.

According to the National Harm Reduction Coalition (NHRC)[1], harm reduction has its roots in many different causes and organizations: The Black Panthers, who started a free breakfast program for children, as well as advocating for healthcare *for all*. These, and other progressive concepts, were designed to not only keep their communities alive but to help them thrive and be the next generation to propel this "radical work" forward, assisting people who have been oppressed for so long.

The Young Lords Organization (YLO) is another group credited for influencing NHRC and spreading harm reduction in the US. Founded in Chicago in 1968, YLO saw its NYC branch create a program of acupuncture for "addicts" living in the Bronx[2]. According to the website of the Museum for the City of New York[3], the Young Lords were a multi-ethnic, Puerto Rican-centered group originating after the garage workers strike in NYC in 1969. Here is more on the group from its website:

It was the summer of 1969, and the group had blocked traffic on 110th Street with piles of garbage to protest inadequate sanitation services. They had already asked the city for brooms to clean their neighborhood's streets and, when refused, they went ahead and took them.

The "garbage offensive" was the first campaign of the city's Young Lords Organization, a radical "sixties" group led by Puerto Rican youth, African Americans, and Latinx New Yorkers. New York's Young Lords, although originally part of a national organization, reflected the lived experiences of Puerto Ricans in New York City. The group mounted eye-catching direct action campaigns against inequality and poverty in East Harlem, the South Bronx, and elsewhere.[4]

Other groups of repressed peoples are also seen as foundational to the harm reduction movement for drug users. For example, the drive toward better healthcare for women particularly in sexual health, increasing 2SLGBTQIA+ rights and treatment for queer folx in particular, during the HIV/AIDS epidemic, was also crucial to establishing NHRC values and how we view harm reduction today. These prior activist movements also helped the national harm reduction movement's growth in other areas, such as learning concepts of organizing, ways to motivate others into action, and how to interact with the public—sometimes radically—to gain political and media notice.[5]

These various groups of historically resilient people carried the lessons of their ancestors about harm reduction; it was and is in their blood (though it wasn't called harm reduction then. It was called survival). Groups with a history of being oppressed always know a lot about survival and therefore they have always known harm reduction.

When the late 12 Stepper cum Harm Reductionist and founder of the Black Harm Reduction Network (BHRN, now the National BHRN), Imani Woods[6] wrote, "There's a fire in my house and you're telling me to rearrange my furniture," what did she mean? Imani was speaking about the Black community's general response to her discussion of needle exchange programs (NEPs) back in the late 1980's and early 1990's. Most folks in those communities equated needles with drug use, which had led to devastation and crime, children left to the care of grandparents or others while their addicted parent(s) searched for the illicit drug they so desperately needed. How were clean needles going to help these problems, they asked? In fact, wouldn't that make illicit IV drug use easier? Many folks in these communities already believed that the government was infiltrating Black communities and distributing crack in order to finally control or eradicate Black populations in urban areas. And no part of any Black community needed more genocide!

Imani says she first encountered the concept of drug-centered harm reduction while studying at the Narcotic and Drug Research Institute in NYC. However, the actual term "harm reduction" wasn't used until Liverpool, England, native Allan Parry came to this country and began to share what England was doing concerning drug use. It was also at the Institute that Imani met Edith Springer, where says she took "every class Edith offered." She really liked Edith's style in trainings but still believed that needle exchange was wrong. However, Imani also states she never encountered an actual needle exchange program until she moved to Seattle in late 1989, following the loss a good friend to AIDS, a friend who was, ironically, vehemently opposed to needle exchange.

Here I'll ask you to come with me as we step back to look at a bit of history in order to better gain perspective on the complex views many in the Black communities were having regarding NEPs and how specifically drug harm reduction—the British/white version—was being received that they were hearing about from mainly whites. And let me be honest here: I needed to be invited to view this perspective from a good friend since I discovered I was making the same mistake as many other white people: assuming BIPOC and other excluded groups were "fearful" of harm reduction. They weren't *fearful*. They knew harm reduction; hell, they *invented* harm reduction just by living their daily lives. They didn't need someone from Liverpool or anywhere else to tell them about how to survive! As that good friend said to me, "The last time the Brits brought us something, it didn't turn out so well." Indeed. So, what *was* going on?

To borrow a phrase … it's complicated. In her chapter in the late professor and researcher G. Alan Marlatt's seminal book *Harm Reduction*[7], Imani talks about how she would go into various Black communities to talk about (drug) harm reduction and how folks were not pleased to hear her. As Imani puts it, they accused her of "bargaining with the Devil." Drug harm reduction and NEPs were not easy conversations to have with anyone back in the mid-late1990's! Remember this was during some of the worst years of the HIV/AIDS epidemic here in the US, when we were just beginning to understand that in order to treat those diseases, we absolutely had to distribute clean needles to IV drug users due to rising transmission rates, especially among Black men. But how was this going to happen in those same Black communities, to be carried out by governmental agencies when those very institutions, especially the bureaucratic healthcare systems, had never bothered to earn this community's trust? Well maybe we need to be asking, "What did we—the majority culture's governmental agencies—do so wrong in these communities?"

There are many examples but let's first look at two big ones. Most of us have heard something about our past government's disgraceful use of Black bodies in medical treatments, such as the infamous Tuskegee syphilis experiment[8] or Henrietta

Lacks[9] stolen cervical cells (which are still in use today). These experiments were done without consent, without knowledge and without consideration of the harms that would likely happen as a result of these tests. In the case of Henrietta Lacks, her cells have been used for decades and have led to amazing discoveries to help millions[10] but her exploitation at the hands of the healthcare system and beyond was mostly unknown by the public until her family successfully sued a biotech company for their continued use of those cells without compensation.

We could also look at how pain has been treated in American Black people. For decades doctors believed that Blacks did not feel pain at the same level as others, thereby denying them the care they needed and should've expected from medical professionals. Even worse, many of these patients were often gaslighted, ignored when they informed medical staff that they were in horrible pain, often due to old myths about the differences of Black bodies from whites[11]. In fact, "40% of first- and second-year medical students endorsed the belief that "black people's skin is thicker than white people's[12].""

Sickle cell anemia[13] is a disease found primarily in those of African descent, though it is also found in some other ethnic groups. The main symptom of this disease is debilitating pain, which can lead to days of excruciating discomfort and agony. Can you imagine being told that you don't need pain medication while you are barely able to breathe? We know that untreated pain leads to added stress, which increases pain. This stress cycle then reduces life spans and quality of life, impairs cognitive abilities, causes hypertension and other heart ailments, and more[14].

For more examples, we could look at how governmental agencies allowed the discriminatory practice known as "red lining" to deny Blacks housing; or how we incarcerate Blacks for drug use at a far higher rate than whites, which often leads to even worse unemployment rates, thus contributing directly to higher rates of problematic drug use. What a circle! Black families also suffered dislocation, including the loss of their homes and property, which happened at a higher rate than it did whites for the same illicit drug use patterns. Mainstream media also needs to take some credit for the distribution of the many myths surrounding drug use and Black people, such as the myth of the "crack baby."[15] What wasn't exaggerated was the level of premeditated violence seen during these "crack" years, which further tore Black communities apart. No wonder when Imani came through talking about clean needles and condoms to reduce harm to suffering communities, many dismissed her as clueless at best and at worst accused her of cavorting with the enemy!

Lastly and perhaps most importantly, what we white folks haven't done much in any community except our own majority white culture is this: *ask folks what they need, ask them how we can help*. Perhaps, with permission from those in the communities, we could share some things that we've discovered help our communities and then ask them, "What do *you* think? Could this possibly help *your* people?" And if they say, "Thanks but no thanks?" Then honor that and shut up. But don't go away mad or insulted. It's just that *every community should have the right to determine what happens to them just like very individual should*. Every group also has a right to be included in any decisions made "for their benefit" (which we'll discuss more in a moment). Remember, sometimes and maybe more often than that, what we think is best for another person or group is in fact exactly wrong for them. Writing all this and reading more on these subjects has also made me wonder if we white folks, the majority culture here in the US, have ever asked another group of even our own nonwhite citizens, *"What's worked for you/your community that we might try with our folks?"*

I keep hearing from Black harm reduction leaders such as Dr. Lisa Moore, Associate Professor of Public Health at SFSU, Joy Rucker, co-founder of the Black Harm Reduction Network (BHRN), Monique Tula, Founder and Principal at Cadence Coaching,[16] and Kassandra Frederique from Drug Policy Alliance[17], and many others, that we must make sure we center the voices (and privilege) of those who use drugs more than those who don't, especially in Black communities. Yes, they are speaking of drug use in the present tense (though we with *lived experience* also have a voice in this discourse, just not as loud or important as those with *living experience*). This makes sense to me as a recovered person: my previous use and various interactions might benefit others, but I have zero personal experience with today's drugs, which are very different from those of past decades. Therefore, treatment and current policies should also look different and be shaped mainly by those with *living experience*. We, with past experience, along with researchers, practitioners, and others, can help guide policies and organizations in viewing historically what's worked, what hasn't, and what things we need to change—valuable learned lessons from our personal (and the country's) past experiences.

Also stated by leaders within Black communities' harm reduction is the need to include Black people when discussing everything about it, from how to speak about harm reduction to the language used. Equally important, we must support the idea of "nothing about us without us," first championed by the disabled community in the 1990's, and often borrowed by other communities seeking visibility and human rights, including the Black communities of harm reductionists. I first heard the phrase while having the honor of working on a grant for African American women's drug treatment services, providing trainings in mainly Motivational Interviewing. I had the privilege to meet (and work with a bit) the Black leader and co-founder of the organization that has adopted its name, *Nothing About Us Without Us*, Dorsey Nunn[18] from that phrase. Strangely, that slogan is believed to have originated in Central Europe—in Latin—to establish foreign policy and legislation. However, it was popularized here in the 1990's by James Charlton, who borrowed it from South African disability activists.[19]

Some may ask, "Where is the proof of the racism and targeting especially of Black drug users?" We acknowledge other minority groups have also been (and continue to be) targets of bias against PWUD but not at the rates Black Americans, who are incarcerated nationally 13 times more than white drug users[20]. But to answer that initial question we need only to look at the history of Black entertainers such as Billie Holliday, a legendary singer so persecuted she ultimately died from an overdose directly due to the prejudices of Harry Anslinger[21], the notorious Commissioner of the US Treasury Department's Federal Bureau of Narcotics.[22] Anslinger staunchly believed that all drugs, save alcohol, should be illegal and was a proponent of campaigns to smear immigrants and various racial groups, making up stories of their drug use to instill fear and hatred in the minds of everyday Americans. The Department was also the forerunner of the current Drug Enforcement Agency (DEA), which is now running a misguided campaign against prescription opiates. Taking a page from Anslinger's book, the DEA is persecuting medical doctors at an alarming rate to curry favor with the public and appear as if they are actively engaged in reducing illicit opiate-related deaths here in America. Sadly, like Anslinger's efforts, none of these measures are based in real science nor are they making any real difference in reducing the rates of substance use disorders or overdoses. They are only succeeding in making sure those pre-scribing doctors and chronic pain patients (which includes Joe and me, and millions of other Americans) suffer needlessly.

We could also look at a 20th century version of racist thinking by examining policies enacted under former President Richard Nix-on. As the originator of our current War on Drugs in 1971, Nixon (who in 1994 was "outted" by his former domestic policy advisor and co-conspirator of the Watergate crimes, John Ehrlichman) apparently lied about his motives as well, just like Anslinger. Quoted here in an April 2016 article by journalist Dan Baum in the magazine *Harper's*[23], Ehrlichman tells us the real story:

The Nixon campaign in 1968, and the Nixon White House after that, had two enemies: the antiwar left and black people," for-mer Nixon domestic policy chief John Ehrlichman told Harper's writer Dan Baum for the April cover story published Tuesday.

"You understand what I'm saying? We knew we couldn't make it illegal to be either against the war or black, but by getting the public to associate the hippies with marijuana and blacks with heroin. And then criminalizing both heavily, we could disrupt those communities," Ehrlichman said. "We could arrest their leaders, raid their homes, break up their meetings, and vilify them night after night on the evening news. Did we know we were lying about the drugs? Of course we did."

55

Clearly I could write forever on the incredible tapestry that is the multi-layered *origins* of harm reduction (and we haven't even touched on valuable harm reduction laws for the non-drug using part of all society, such as seat belts in cars, motorcycle helmets, and the like) and on the racist drug laws we still have, but many great writers have already done that. Thankfully, many journalists and writers continue to examine our unscientific drug laws and advocate for changes too. I invite you to research these topics yourselves. (I will post a few books on my website to get you started once this book is launched, though you can also find several in the endnotes in this book. I myself wouldn't have known as much about these topics—of which I continue to learn constantly—if I hadn't taught courses on Drugs and Society and Public Policy for two decades.)

To close this chapter, let me once again invoke the Spirit of Imani Woods and quote her words: "...without a working knowledge of Black culture, respect for the Black agenda, and appreciation of the complexities involved, any harm reduction endeavor targeting the Black community will fail."[24] While she was writing in 1998, her comments still ring true today, perhaps more than ever. We can and must do better for all drug users and their families/loved ones and especially for Black Americans and all the many other persons and communities living in the shadow of the majority white culture. At its core, harm reduction is about saving lives—*all* lives. Much like the Jewish saying that opens this chapter, we believe that each human being is worth saving and that doing so ultimately saves all of us. In order to accomplish this task, we must therefore make room for all in the harm reduction movement in order to stay true to our roots as advocates, mavericks, and shit disturbers—if we are truly to *meet people where they are and not leave them there*, including those who are not yet part of our movement. We may not agree on all the policies or politics of harm reduction, nor even its history, but there is no other way forward if we are truly to make "any positive change"[25] possible.

This chapter is dedicated to all the poor white Punks, the Disabled, Indigenous, Black, Brown, Person of Color, Queer, Immigrant—anyone who has ever been excluded from the majority culture for being who they are.

Endnotes

1.https://harmreduction.org/movement/evolution/. Accessed 11.24.2024

2. https://www.curbed.com/2021/10/young-lords-acupuncture-detox-bronx-lincoln-hospital.html

3. https://www.mcny.org/exhibition/young-lords

4. Ibid

5. https://harmreduction.org/movement/evolution/. Accessed 11.24.2024

6. Imani Woods died in 2015. She was also a founder member of the Harm Reduction Coalition & ED of SOS harm reduction programs in Seattle, WA. May she continue to Rest in Power

7. Marlatt, G.A. (1998) Harm Reduction. The Guilford Press. NY, NY

8. https://eji.org/news/history-racial-injustice-tuskegee-syphilis-experiment/

9. https://www.bbc.com/news/world-us-canada-66376758

10. https://apnews.com/article/henrietta-lacks-hela-cells-thermo-fisher-scientific-bfba4a6c10396efa34c9b79a544f0729

11. https://www.aamc.org/news/how-we-fail-black-patients-pain

12. Ibid

13. https://www.cdc.gov/sickle-cell/complications/pain.html#:~:-text=Pain%20is%20the%20most%20common,throughout%20the%20body%2C%20causing%20pain

14. https://www.curepain.net/blog/8-serious-health-complications-of-untreated-chronic-pain#:~:text=The%20longer%20you%20spend%20in,in%20the%20most%20severe%20cases

15. https://www.npr.org/2010/05/03/126478643/crack-babies-twenty-years-later; https://www.brown.edu/Administration/News_Bureau/2003-04/03-099.html#:~:text=The%20term%20%E2%80%9Ccrack%20baby%E2%80%9D%20is,desperately%20in%20need%20of%20care

16. https://www.cadenceconsulting.community/

17. https://drugpolicy.org/person/kassandra-frederique/

18. https://www.instagram.com/anewwayoflifela/p/C8-ZEBCgNgd/

19. https://philadelphia.center.psu.edu/news/nothing-about-us-without-us-introduction-to-participatory-action-research/#:~:text=The%20

mantra%20likely%20originated%20in,from%20South%20African%20disability%20activists

20. https://www.hrw.org/legacy/campaigns/drugs/war/key-facts.htm#:~:-text=Nationwide%2C%20blacks%20comprise%2062%20percent,the%20rate%20of%20white%20men. Accessed 11.24.24

21. According to journalist Johann Hari, the Federal Bureau of Narcotics under Anslinger targeted Billie Holiday in response to her 1939 song "Strange Fruit," which criticized racist lynchings. Hari wrote that Anslinger assigned an agent to track her after she refused to stop speaking out about racism

22. Anslinger served for an unprecedented 32 years, under the presidencies of Herbert Hoover, Franklin D. Roosevelt, Harry S. Truman, Dwight D. Eisenhower, and John F. Kennedy. https://en.wikipedia.org/wiki/Harry_J._Anslinger

23. https://harpers.org/archive/2016/04/legalize-it-all/

24. Marlatt, G.A. (1998) Harm Reduction. The Guilford Press. NY, NY. p322

25. Quote from the late Dan Bigg, co-founder of the Chicago Recovery Alliance (CRA)

PART 1

POLICY/ADVOCATES & PEOPLE WHO USE/
USED DRUGS (PWUD)

BRIAN BOURASSA

I was in my third year of living outside, the last year of being homeless, and I had been living up at the Russian River area in the woods, and I finally got my SSDI (Social Security Disability Insurance) benefits. So, I decided to come back to the City (San Francisco) and get back into doing something seriously. I was out on 6th Street one day and I saw a place, a needle exchange, where you could go and get clean drug using supplies. And they had coffee. They also had testing for STDs, information on housing, food, treatment … all kinds of stuff. And you know, I just kept showing up regularly to that needle exchange. One day, this lady named Terry Morris took me aside and said, "Hey, I have this book club on Mondays called *Over the Influence*. It's a harm reduction book club so you can come how you want to come." She continued, "If you want to come and sleep during the whole hour, you can sit in your chair and sleep; you just can't be disruptive. And I make a killer keg of coffee so you can have all the coffee you want." But she went even further: "What would you say if I told you that there's a way to keep yourself in really good health, like you've been doing by coming here, and while you're in active addiction? We have all these different tracks that you can try with no judg-ment. And you can manage your health a lot better, get some clarity around your addiction and stuff. What do you think?" And I said, "Okay." That was my invitation to the book club and harm reduction.

The book club was held at the San Francisco AIDS Foundation. It was part of their Stonewall Project. They had all these harm re-duction programs, I guess you could call them different recovery programs—outpatient recovery tracks that were all under this harm reduction "umbrella." I started going on Mondays and I really loved the book! We would read part of it and then discuss it. It was great. Terry was the first person that I ever felt was really open to people talking about their weekend, about using drugs, everything. It wasn't about glorifying drug use either. It was just like, "This is what I did this weekend, and I feel horrible today," or "I feel really good—I only used this weekend." I started learning not only from her, but from my peers in the room—how people move through life and their ad-diction, but not chastise themselves or try to make themselves feel bad about it. Just accepting that, "This is where I am in my life right now. I don't know if I'm going to be here forever. But I understand who I am as an addict." And that's what drew me to harm reduction.

To me, harm reduction means taking care of yourself while you're in active addiction so that if and when you do decide to get clean, you haven't really torn yourself up. You know, there's a lot of stuff out there that you can get besides HIV—there's hepa-titis C, and that lives *outside* the body. If you are an IV drug user, which I was on occasion, there's a lot of fear around getting Hep C. I didn't know a lot about it back then, but I would never share needles anyway because I'm HIV positive. But sometimes you're in a certain state of mind and a lot of the things you don't typically do, you wind up doing. Being in the harm reduction program was always a constant reminder that it's okay if you're using but you need to be using in a responsible way—for the safety of yourself and others. That's what that program and harm reduction really taught me—to take better care of myself.

A lot of their literature and services are geared towards things like, "Are you paranoid? Well, you might be paranoid because you need to get more sleep. You've been up for four days," and I'm like, "Oh, *that's* why I'm paranoid." I learned maybe it isn't the drugs. Maybe I'm paranoid because I haven't had sleep in four nights, and that's all I need to do. Or maybe I need to check that I've eaten today, or maybe I need to drink more water. The program literature might ask, "Are you at least drinking Ensure?" I learned to do that all the time, just to keep weight on me when I was using meth because I would lose so much weight that I couldn't eat. I learned about these basic techniques that you could do to sustain weight so your body wasn't just getting eaten away. It helped avoid things like infections. I learned a much better way to take care of myself and where I was in my addiction.

I wish people understood more about harm reduction! It's a perfectly viable way of recovering. When people decide to do the AA program for instance, they lock into that, and it can really work for them. Maybe they've tried other methods, and finally something about that program sticks. So, they lock into it, and they hold on to it for dear life. And that's great for them. But sometimes I feel these folks can get a little judgmental—just because that's working for them does not mean that there aren't other viable recovery programs out there that can work for others. We also need to talk more about if AA or other 12 Step programs don't work for you, how it doesn't mean you're weak, or you're a "cop out," or that you're not taking your recovery seriously—all things I heard at times when I went to 12 Step meetings. And those are not things I ever heard while being in a harm reduction program.

Today, I am a staunch harm reductionist. If anybody asks me, I'll tell them, "I do harm reduction to this very day. I'm very proud of that. Harm reduction saved my life. It kept me alive. And it kept me healthy while I was trying to recover." It was a harm reduction group that really showed up for me when I was trying to quit meth and recover—and when I really started to infuse it into my life. I tell people that in harm reduction, there's also an abstinence track—there's many tracks, like a partial abstinence, or a substance replacement track. For instance, let's say you're doing meth and you decide, "I'm going to give this up and I'm just going to smoke weed. Weed is going to be my thing." In a harm reduction track, that's totally great. I know people who did that. They went to AA because they were raging alcoholics, but they called me up and said, "Hey, I'm in AA but I'm doing edibles. What do you think?" And I said, "Well, you need to talk to your sponsor first because AA can be all or nothing. But, look, have you relapsed in the two months that you stopped drinking alcohol? No? Well, obviously, weed isn't a trigger." That's how I would look at it. If you're relapsing and picking up a cocktail whenever you smoke weed, then you might want to look at that; weed might be a trigger. I'm very lucky. The only trigger that I had in my life was sex sites. That's where I got introduced to meth—for the second time in my life. So, I have to stay away from all online dating apps, everything. As long as I steer clear of those, I'm totally fine.

I even found that I can have a drink, though I'm not drinking right now. I decided to do a "harm reduction experiment" at the beginning of the year and stop drinking for three months. I was surprised that I had a two-week detox, but I had been drinking a lot. I successfully stopped drinking for three months. And then in the fourth month, after I started drinking again, I decided, "I'm gonna try this again." And you know what? I noticed that I had definitely cut back. I wasn't drinking like I was before, but I also noticed that alcohol just wasn't feeling right for me anymore. Like it wasn't feeling the same. And so, after doing it for three months, I stopped again. It's been six weeks and I just the other day said, "You know what, I think it's time to give up alcohol. It's not working for me. I don't like the way it's making me feel." There you go. Harm reduction is working in my life again, in a different way.

My experiences, as well as watching others around me, have led me to believe that harm reduction should be more at the forefront of all recovery. I see it from the perspective of a person recovering. I'm here in Hawaii and I see how crystal meth has affected the community here. I see it on the street (I can spot a tweaker a mile away because I used to be one). And I don't think there's a lot of harm reduction here. At least I'm not hearing harm reduction in the dialogue sadly. I haven't been to many AA meetings or such, but I have met people in recovery here. It's just interesting because I can see that harm reduction would be so helpful here in Hawaii.

Harm reduction has gotten a lot of legitimization over the last few years. I knew about it back in 2013 and it was already kind of going strong before that, but it had to be done in a very secret way back then. In fact, at the SF AIDS Foundation they have the original baby buggy that workers used to put clean syringes and other supplies in and distribute them out on the streets. We need to never go back to that. We need to move forward with harm reduction, which is why I'd like to see it come out from the underground, to be right in the forefront of recovery, everywhere.

The last thing I'll say about harm reduction is this: when I originally began attending that harm reduction program at the Foundation, I started with a group of men who are all friends. One of them is my friend "Kyle." He and all the other fellas in that little group of friends relapsed. They had gotten clean together using both 12 Step and attending the harm reduction group, and they managed to stay clean for a while. And then, one by one, they all relapsed. Coming out of that last relapse seemed really hard for all of them but especially for Kyle. One of the things I noticed was that when they went back to AA or NA to try to clean up again, they were given a lot of flak about relapsing and being away from the groups. They were definitely chronic relapsers, but they weren't getting any understanding or support in their 12 Step groups, which just made it harder for these guys [to get help]. But in the harm reduction group, nobody was judging them, so they really took that group and our support to heart. This last time when they went back to AA they were able to say, "Hey, wait a minute, this harm reduction program is also viable, it's helpful, and it kept me alive. And now I'm back in the rooms so you can't discount that."

I saw these conversations about harm reduction really start to happen a lot in 12 Step meetings! For instance, I heard the conversations change at the Castro Country Club, which was a big 12 Step meeting place. I heard people talking about harm reduction all over the Castro, and I would love to see more of that dialogue. I think it's important and it's time. Any of us can get tunnel vision and say, "Oh, this is the only way to recover," or we can be open to other ways, other paths. And 12 Step asks us to be "honest, open minded, and willing." That's how we evolve, that's how we grow as a society. It's scary, sure, but you have to do it. I had to do it to recover and my life here is so blessed today I can hardly believe it. It really can happen, and it takes all paths. And to me, that's harm reduction.

Brian Bourassa can be reached at 1313nmarrs@gmail.com @bb_tree67 (IG)

JOE CLIFFORD

I came to harm reduction is a roundabout way. In fact, at the time, I thought I discovered it! This is less about hubris or my being a visionary than it speaks to my stubbornness, which was equally matched by the recovery industry at the time when I was trying to get straight.

Talking about this time of my life, my period of "active addiction" for lack of a better word, I've grown, I don't want to say "weary," because it's an important subject, i.e., showing change is possible and all that, but I wrote a book about it. Literally. Or literarily. And that's not to move copies. You get a little worn down discussing the same thing over.

Since that book (*Junkie Love*), I've written almost two dozen more, but any interview I give, however recent a release I'm promoting, somehow, we always come back to this topic. I get it. The ten years I spent homeless and addicted in San Francisco in the '90s *is* the sexier story. The nuts and bolts about *how* I did it get glossed over. Time is limited. It's nice to be able to share my story—my *full* story, or at least as much as I can squeeze in over a couple thousand words!

When I was finally done with that life, I checked myself into a long-term treatment facility for six months, and returned to school, earned my degree, got married (and quickly divorced), earned another degree, remarried, published books, had kids and all the rest (including divorced again), and now I'm helping put out a second edition on harm reduction.

I am also a professor at Florida International Universal, have edited numerous publications, and published even more books.

This introduction is about as whittled down as I can get it.

In between those two timelines (the drug use and my return to functional society), there was a *lot* of what AA might call "failed attempts." In all, I went to rehab around twenty times. And before I am critical of AA or 12 Step programs, I want to say that I am only able to offer this insight, i.e., am not dead or, worse, in prison, because of the generosity of the recovery/re-hab communities, *including* AA, the hospitals and drunk tanks and state-paid psychiatrists and myriad assorted "welfare" doctors. I can't heap enough praise on the kindness of these strangers, men and woman who will *never know* the impact they made. If it wasn't for the whole "anonymity" thing, I'd be impelled to share each and every one of their names, because I remember them. I remember each time they took me aside and offered words of encouragement, displayed much needed compassion, and helped hold me up long enough till I was able to finally stand on my own.

Almost invariably these same folks were operating from the dark, telling me the only way out was to attend meetings. And in the words of my former writing professor, the late Dan Wake-field (*New York in the Fifties*), "Yeah, AA helped me quit. I knew if I didn't quit I'd have to go to those fucking meetings." Without knowing it, I was also practicing harm reduction. Cobbling together fragments of philosophy kept me alive another day until I could figure out what I was doing. Ultimately, hardheaded with an iron will, I *had* to do it *my* way. And *that's* harm reduction: meeting the client where they are *at that moment.*

Drinking was never my problem. It wasn't until a few years ago I cut out alcohol entirely. I stopped the hard drugs in 2002, but would periodically drink, socially. It wasn't until the death of my brother and the pandemic, that "socially" became a little more, and then I stopped. Wasn't a big deal. Quitting drinking was like taking new vitamins for me, or any other mundane change. That's because I'd already done the *hardest* thing I've ever done in my life when I quit heroin, meth, and cocaine almost twenty years earlier. After *that*? You can quit damn never anything, with ease.

But to go back to that part I glossed over, the "how" I quit heroin and stopped being homeless and living "a life of crime" was anything but a straight line. And despite the good hearts of so many in the rehab/recovery community, I could not, or to go full Dr. Suess, cannot, will not, have not, and never will, be part of 12 Steps. I was what they called in Chapter Five that person "incapable of being honest." I'm paraphrasing, using their words, because I sure as shit ain't opening that damned book again.

Like I said, I'm hardheaded. Was then, am now. I am not always easy to be around (just ask my latest ex-wife), but I'm also not full of shit. I grew up Christian, and though I still tick that box on official forms, my God is a God of one, for me and *only* me, and for all the AA/NA proselytizing how the "Higher Power" could be anything you want ("It can be a doorknob!" "A lightbulb!"), when you close with the Lord's Prayer, it's a Christian program. And though I might identify as a Christian, I don't agree with 99.9% of others who do. (I won't bring politics into this. Leave it at: I am so left of center, my hats border blue to black.)

While harm reduction was saving my life, I didn't know it was called that at the time. I knew the road I was headed down wasn't a good one and that it was time for a major change. I was "sick and tired of being sick and tired," but I never wanted to stop being *me*. Being true to oneself is, for me, the highest peak one can strive for. I didn't want to hate myself or *every-thing* I believed in. I wanted to extrapolate the "junkie" part of me and continue on. I was told, point blank, that simply wasn't possible. I needed to be broken. Like I was a wild stallion or something.

When I was getting straight, there was one ticket out: 12 Steps. Get a sponsor, work the steps, go to those fucking meetings, and I said no. So, of course, each time I fell short, I was told, "Well, obviously, you didn't work the steps!" But, they'd add, "feel free to go back out and try it your way, Joe." So I did.

Eighteen trips back and forth, in and out of rehab, until I did what I was told was impossible: I got straightened out through force of will.

Which is how I viewed it for many years, fostering more animosity toward the faceless, nameless recovery industry. I thought I'd bucked the system, a renegade. Until I was introduced to the term "harm reduction." Which is when I realized I'd been practicing its tenets the entire time! And had a lot of help from advocates of its principles.

Before my writing started taking off, I returned to school to get my drug and alcohol certification. I wanted to offer what so many had offered me, but I wanted to do so without the guise of 12 Steps. (I never got that certification because the books took off. One of the *best* parts about the success of *Junkie Love*—also one of the most heartbreaking parts—is the chance I get to discuss the truth about recovery with the wives, mothers, fathers, husbands, sisters, and brothers of addicts, as well drug users themselves. I get lots of email from folks wanting to talk about the book, and I hear their stories, and we get to have one-on-one communication about the grim realities of drug use. But those conversation also, invariably, show hope is always possible.)

In these classes, I started to realize that, no, I didn't do it through will power alone. Yes, I had a *very* spiteful streak, and I used this rather "negative" emotion to fuel what was, in reality, an imaginary fight toward a better end. But as I mentioned, I had *a lot* of assistance along the way. And while I rejected AA/NA steadfastly, and found the meetings to be, at best, hellish, I *was* benefitting in other ways from my "failed" attempts.

I lived in a city where 99% of intravenous users had HIV and/or Hep C. I was careful, sure, but I also can't take credit for being *that* lucky (which is how I made peace with my *own* God). Moreover, there were practical applications at every stop. Access to clean needles (harm reduction). Money for my blood to get tested (harm reduction). I get twenty dollars, we were able to see if I remained disease free, *and* that's one fix I didn't have to steal for. The soup kitchens. The rehabs themselves. There was one place that would travel *anywhere* in New England to pick you up and bring you to their facility, free of charge. Though I lived in San Francisco, I was from the East Coast, where my brother still lived; I was, in large part, a drifter. That was *huge*. Pick up a payphone (I'm dating myself) and call an 800 number, and they'd send someone to the depths of Nordic hell and bring me somewhere safe. These are *all* examples of harm reduction.

Each time, I was getting a little bit better.

I still fought against AA and its purveyors and minions. But I was *also* learning that there was another way out. For me, in retrospect, I was practicing, benefiting from, and now promote all these aspects of harm reduction.

When people ask me what "harm reduction" means now, I put in the simplest terms. For me, it means, "If you're getting high/drunk/living an unstable existence seven days a week, let's see if we can get that down to six." I'm oversimplifying, but they usually get the point. Or in the words of the great Australian singer/songwriter Paul Kelly, "If drinking is the problem, drink a little less."

It is wonderful—absolutely-fucking-wonderful—if someone can and *wants* to be abstinent, and if in doing so, they are able to live their *best* life, however they define it. There is also, for me, a lot of room in the middle. To me, that's where harm reduction's future enters the conversation: people who use aren't stupid, so let's stop the bullshit, eh?

We are a chemical culture. Whether that's the state-sanctioned alcohol or newly legalized weed, or laudanum from the 1880s. That's the funny thing with drugs—*any* drug: it's always okay if you do the drugs *they* do. Drink an evening glass of wine and smoke some weed? Sure. But, no, you shouldn't be on opiate-based painkillers (even if they are prescribed by doctors, aware of your situation, and you *must* take them after you broke half your bones in a motorcycle accident—I might be projecting on that last one!). My point: I know very, very few people who live 100% substance free. They just qualify it, rearranging morality to make permissible the drugs *they* take, while vilifying the ones *you* take.

This is the hypocrisy I saw in rehabs. This was the impossible standard I saw "in the rooms," where many times addictions were swapped out for standing around in a circle, thanking Jesus, two hours a day for the rest of your life, and drinking burnt coffee as you looking down on the lesser-thans. Again, that works for *you*, God bless.

It didn't for me. It didn't for *a lot* of users I knew. And instead of being offered alternatives, we were blamed. (There's a cartoon I love. There's an old man with his wife at a funeral. He looks over the body in the casket and says to his wife, "I told Bob he'd die without AA. Took forty years. But he finally proved me right." Ha!)

I couldn't buy into 12 Steps because I can't believe in a God who would grant me intelligence and then punish me for using it. I *could* buy into (can and will continue to buy into) harm reduction. Narcan, methadone, food, clothing, shelter, empathy, helping however one can, and stopping with the Puritanical judgment when someone fails to live up to *your* standards.

So much of this comes down to rewording.

Though I despise much of AA, I do *love* their bumper stickers.

In the end, AA and harm reduction intersect on one vital, undeniable point: Don't give up until the miracle happens. Getting wasted every day was the solution for an angry 23-year-old boy. It doesn't work for a ~~53-year-old~~ 54-year-old man.

I see humor in darkness. I laugh at the morbid, as I endure the losses of those closest to me, like my brother, Josh, who simply couldn't make it out and join me. I've retained a lot of anger, which I use to push myself to be the best version of myself (which isn't for everybody).

To get here? I needed to stay alive long enough for that to happen.

That's harm reduction.

Joe can be reached at joe@joeclifford.com

LAURA GUZMAN

I came to harm reduction by "accident," although in retrospect I was exactly where I was supposed to be in 1995. It happened that I finished law school, did not pass the California bar (my death penalty), my law school internship as an investigator ended, and I needed a job as a single momma to support our family. Twenty-nine years ago, I got hired at AIDS Benefits Counselors (ABC) in San Francisco as a bilingual, outreach benefits advocate. I had worked a summer at Solano County Legal Aid, in Vallejo, California, where I learned to represent Black and Brown elders who were not receiving SSI (even though they should have been) and was trained by a super sassy and talented Puerto Rican paralegal sister who sang *boleros* and salsa songs. At ABC, my role was to advocate and provide access to income and Medi-Cal benefits to people diagnosed with AIDS who were neglected and stigmatized for using and injecting drugs, for being queer and trans, for being Black, Brown, and poor. I was invited to rotate outreach services in the Tenderloin and was stationed two days a week at the Ambassador Hotel, where I learned quickly and so much, and across the City (San Francisco) where I supported poor people living with HIV/AIDS on their SSI/MediCal journey. That is when and how my harm reduction voyage started.

I learned from harm reduction pioneers in the City, including nurses, social workers and people living and dying from AIDS, and people who used drugs, including heroin and meth injectors. I joined the first harm reduction working groups in San Francisco, led by amazing humans like super nurse Diane Jones, who worked for Visiting Nurses and Hospices and was one of the first attending to people dying of AIDS at Ward 86. I quickly learned that in doing front line work in the belly of the beast, my service and advocacy were inseparable [to bring forth] social justice and change. Before I left Argentina ten years prior, I was a youth socialist organizer, who worked to end the bloodiest military dictatorship and fought for an anti-imperialist, loving, and liberated world. The concept: harm reduction was liberatory. In learning about its principles and loving practices that elevated the active participation and needs of PWUD (people who use drugs) in their health and overall wellbeing, made total sense to me and became a mission and my passion. Here I am, twenty-nine years later, still focused on this work, which I believe requires us to act selflessly, to love ourselves deeply, and to collectively push towards the liberation of ourselves, our people, and each other—a high call.

Although we often say that "harm reduction is love," we forget to practice love with ourselves. So here I am in my life trajectory, almost sixty years old, making self-love a daily discipline, a practice with a *bunch* of things that I need to remember: taking my medication so my cholesterol is not so high; grounding practices and microdosing so my high anxiety is reduced; taking herbs to diminish the impact of menopause; watching what

I eat; and trying to create space for breathing and moving my body—while working remotely fifty hours or so a week. What I am finding is that the more I practice, the more that I remember to do these healthier things. The more I manifest loving myself, first, it helps me prioritize my time and say, "No, I don't want to spend it doing this (or that)." And this is *all* harm reduction! I am continuously inspired by this idea that if we think about love for ourselves, harm reduction requires us to really keep practicing again and again, one thing at a time.

I also like connecting harm reduction (and all my work in community) with the Buddhist concept of a Bodhisattva, the one that stays until the end to save others in the saga of the Buddha or particularly in the tradition of Tibetan Buddhism. Buddhist nun Pema Chodron talks about the Bodhisattva way. The Bodhisattva personifies one that is selfless, they will do whatever it takes to save others. And they wind up, in some ways, saving themselves. I love that tradition. And I love the concept of giving and selflessness because there is a lot of that in harm reduction, although at times to the detriment of ourselves. There is something fundamental and beautiful about selflessness, which makes people truly courageous. I see the Bodhisattva really represents that kind of quality and harm reduction, no matter where we work: frontlines, advocacy, policy, research, or somewhere else in harm reduction. We may be further from the frontlines but that does not mean we may not still be a Bodhisattva. That does not mean we still do not sacrifice, but it is a different level of sacrifice. It requires continued, sustained effort and love for the people.

As a new national leader at NHRC, and someone who worked in the trenches for three decades, I am paying attention to the organizations and fields in which we have not partnered yet closely enough, and where it is important we infuse our harm reduction framework and set of proven practices to support people who use drugs; we continue to elevate drug user health through capacity building and advocacy efforts in working to address the very drivers of inequality, such as racism and the War on Drugs, mass incarceration, militarism and colonial and imperial wars spending, and the decimation of critical safety nets and affordable housing, among others.

This is particularly relevant, given that in the last few years we have witnessed a sudden 360 degree turn towards and against harm reduction (a weird dichotomy) fueled by our broken systems of care and failed policies before and after Covid, including mass uprisings calling for racial justice after police murders of Black and Brown folks across the country, calls to defund police, the deepening of the income divide and growth of health and housing inequities, the growing rate of overdose deaths in communities of color, a tainted drug supply, and as we (deal with) national elections, politicians return to "law and order" and criminalization efforts on the back of our communities, to gain votes and legitimize existing harmful power structures.

I have been involved in the National Healthcare for the Homeless movement for a long time because the clinic I ran in the Mission district for sixteen years was a homeless clinic within a federally qualified health center. I have also been an HCH community commissioner for Alameda County since 2018. I chose to participate in the HCH movement as a close partner of our work, given that the HCH Council was born in the mid-80's and formed by doctors, nurses, social workers, and homeless advocates who began seeing a growing number of unhoused patients who were not getting the medical care (or housing) they needed and deserved. It has been a true blessing to be in the HCH world and embrace harm reduction, both. I first heard of buprenorphine to treat unhoused patients sometime in 2007 at an HCH National Conference, and two years later, when I visited Albuquerque HCH in my fellowship, one of the first in the country to open an SSP and offer bupe treatment in clinical settings after patients [were] release[d] from jail. We implemented buprenorphine treatment (and referrals to methadone) at my homeless program's clinic a few years later, following these mentor programs. I had the privilege to attend the HCH National Conference right before Covid. I saw the growth of buprenorphine and MAT-focused workshops. I reached out to the Council's CEO, Bobby Watts, and his team, and formed a collaborative partnership with the Council. In 2022 and 2024, we teamed up to offer a harm reduction pre-conference in Baltimore and harm reduction-infused training in Arizona, and now I am seated at their National Board of Directors, ready to continue our partnership to bring forth equity and harm reduction into the field. As over 70% of SSP participants meet the federal definition of homelessness, this allegiance and our future advocacy efforts are key.

I was privileged to be among the first trainers for the Harm Reduction Coalition West Coast Institute in 1999. In the first cohort, I was trained and coached in Oakland's HRC office in the first Train the Trainers (ToT) project, led by fabulosa Edith Springer, one of the most inspiring harm reductionists in the United States, and Alessandra Ross, who is now lead at the California Department of Public Health, Office of AIDS Harm Reduction Unit, and a recent funder of our California work. At the time, the West Coast Institute was led by my wonderful sister Maria Chavez, who was recruiting peeps in the field doing harm reduction work. We were trained in adult education and capacity building skills while supported to incorporate practice, data, and advocacy in our training institute. We were learners and teachers, both, and some of us organizers as well. I had the honor to do my first co-facilitated training for the Institute along with Jeannie Little, founder of HRTI (Harm Reduction Training Institute), as graduates of that first cohort, and did my second "mandatory" harm reduction training on my own in San Jose for a group of "drunk-driving" instructors. Although this was just my second training for HRC, the trainees were not happy they had to undergo training in harm reduction, and given that most of them were people in recovery and believed mostly in abstinence-based approaches, they had little sympathy for "meeting anybody where they were at" in their active drug use. Period.

As I was going through the training, I had a particular audience member, a tall and big, heavily tattooed white instructor, who challenged everything I said. I quickly realized he was not going to have it, and in spite of how nervous I was, I remembered to "meet him where [he] was at," and also follow one of our ToT's advice: "When something gets heated or controversial, open up the discussion, and let the group talk it through facilitated discussion." As I was talking about the need and right to house people who use drugs, my challenger stated, "Why would you waste housing resources on someone who does not care about themselves by using drugs? Why would they have a right to housing?" And then, kinda magically, an elderly, Black instructor stopped him, swiftly, and responded, "She got a point. When I was down and out, if someone would have given me a hand, such as housing, I may not have suffered on the streets so much for so long, as I did." A whole conversation about hitting (or not) rock bottom ensued and the energy was shifted to include housing people when they are "down and out," as a critical service to support their well-being and recovery.

When training was over, the big man got close to me and said, "I still do hate harm reduction, but this was the best harm reduction training I ever attended," and shook my hand and left. I am not sure if I moved him some from where he was (highly likely not) but it felt good to have been acknowledged for facilitating a good training session.

Strategy matters when training on harm reduction, and being ready and willing to be challenged is so important. It takes time to feel comfortable, though, and, with time, I learned that harm reduction teaches us to do that, helping us to remain with a "beginners' mind," to help ourselves and others to get a bit closer to understanding and embracing our principles and actions. What our people hear in the news, on the street and social media may be awful (against harm reduction), and therefore ignorance may be disguised by unintelligent and mean comments. Cueing into the audience, being open to all challenges, and working ourselves to stay grounded and focused, is key to transforming harm reduction work, so we keep pushing the envelope collectively with and for people who use drugs. Doing this work for decades grounded within Black and Brown communities, where our folks' views are not initially too hopeful or maybe folks are not embracing harm reduction for exceptionally good reasons, taught me that. We also need to remember we are both learners and teachers. That makes harm reduction education key, as our roots are not founded in academia but on the streets, where we continuously learn and are advised on what our folks know and need.

And that gets me to remind myself not to get "too stuck" about language, and when I say language, I mean how much we prescribe or condemn how people talk about their own "addiction" and/or substance use, or someone else's drug use. Our folks talk about their complicated relationship with drugs in ways that may not meet "harm reduction academia," harm reduction tenets, or anti-stigmatizing language. To do this work we must always keep it real. I love that we have moved from talking about "drug users" to "people who use drugs." I believe when people use disparaging language, those are real opportunities to learn and teach each other, raise stigma as something that truly gets into our ability to see ourselves changing and taking any positive steps. We can shift the focus from drugs and people who use drugs to emphasize the particular violent conditions in which our people are stigmatized beyond language: the struggle for survival, homelessness, lack of empathy from housed folks and the daily violence exercised against them, the pressure to quit without being ready, willing and able, all of them real markers about how hard it still is for our communities to feel seen, be agents of their own destiny, and having the ability to access spaces to feel safe, to grow and thrive. Language is a part of this equation.

What I like to use for a definition of harm reduction is the development and support of critical services and advocacy to reduce and eliminate drug related harms, broadly, and most importantly, the affirmation of the fundamental human rights of poor people who use drugs, in particular Black, Brown and native folks, trans and queer people, those unhoused, currently and formerly incarcerated, and sex workers. We have to provide access to housing, income, comprehensive health care, treatment and healing options, and freedom from criminalization, which is still the primary default mode to address drug-related harms in this country and abroad. (We need) recognition of people's freedom and autonomy and supports over punishment. Since historically most "drug-related harm" is directly correlated to failed policies and punitive frameworks, working towards human rights and equity and dismantling systems of harm is still the work to be done for our harm reduction futures.

Laura can be reached at guzman@harmreduction.org

TRACEY HELTON

The first time I heard the term "harm reduction," I was an IV drug user in the '90s. I started using around 1990, maybe 1989. We had one syringe that my friends and I all shared. We kept it so long until the syringe looked and felt like an old fish hook. I was so worried I was never gonna get another one.

When I moved to San Francisco, I visited the needle exchange, and learned how much damage I'd done using that same syringe over and over. I remember one point, I could not put my hands down because they would, you know, pulsate with pain—just from using the same syringe. From that point, I'd wait in line each week to get my supply. There wasn't an endless supply, it was a one-to-one exchange, but it had a profound impact on me.

There was a guy in my building—this was around 1992—named Raven, who would go around to the whole building and collect the syringes. And then when I was homeless, I would go around and do the same for other users who were also displaced. That was my introduction to the people working for the syringe exchange, who were very, very nice. That was my introduction to needle exchanges, and really how I learned about harm reduction.

The needle exchange was like the water cooler, a place to gather with other users. You'd find out who was in jail, who in the hospital, who had left town. It kept you connected.

When I went to rehab in 1998, I had started volunteering at this place called the Sage Project, which was a hybrid harm reduction slash abstinence program. The Sage Project also worked with people involved in sex work and sexual exploitation. Often these were teenagers. We'd supply condoms and offer other forms of support.

I gravitated more toward those who used drugs. It's where I felt I could offer the most help. The people who ran Sage asked if I'd participate in a specific group, the SF Heroin Committee. At the time, San Francisco was in the grips of an overdose crisis. During this span, at its peak, we had close to two hundred overdoses in the city, which seems so small compared to today, where that number is closer to seven hundred. There was a very focused effort in the late-'90s to get users and friends and family involved with preventing overdoses.

In 2000, I attended the Heroin Conference in Seattle. Many in the industry—a lot my age—were there to see Dan Bigg's talk advocating naloxone distribution. It was very inspiring, encouraging attendees to bring this approach back to their home states. At the time, my recovery was very much abstinence based. My perspective changed when a friend of mine, who had been on methadone, was convinced by a person in NA to get off it. They told him as long as he was on methadone, he wasn't clean, he wasn't sober. My friend stopped taking methadone, and ended up relapsing and dying. That's when I realized my bias around abstinence wasn't necessarily helpful to others. If I really wanted the best for people, I needed to meet them where they were at, ask what was best for *them* and *their* lives. Maybe that was abstinence. Maybe it was another approach. That's when all different elements of harm reduction came together for me. Recovery encompasses an entire spectrum.

Everyone's experience is different. I was working with a lot of Black and Latino folks, many of whom were working in the various aspects of the sex industry. Of course, I don't want people doing sex work because I had just gotten out. In my very narrow frame, I don't want that for you! But this was survival sex for them. It was about what they wanted or needed to do to support themselves. My experiences and what others faced weren't always going to line up, and I needed to appreciate how other people's experience can be totally different. This was when I began to break off from some of my early teachers. I felt they were stripping folks of their autonomy by imposing a one-size-fits-all mandate. I don't know what another's experiences are. For some, sex work was easier than working in retail. There were others, like members of the trans community, who couldn't get hired at a regular job because of discrimination. So, that was what they were doing; people were using drugs for a variety of reasons. I found it more productive to guide people toward a healthier, happier path than stringently impose *my* way of thinking.

Treatment centers have changed since back in my day. It used to be, you could go in for six months, and when you got out you'd have a soft landing and help reintegrating to society; you'd get help with housing, finding a job. Now, Medicare will pay for two ninety-day stays. Except ... if you go in one day and find you're not getting the help you need and leave? That counts as one [attempt]. I'll meet a lot of people who are like, "Well, that was hell. No one helped me with withdrawal or getting sober. I'm going to be homeless anyway. Why bother?" This can cost someone a year of treatment options. How is that helping?

There used to be Walden House, which used to have its own secondary housing. This approach was fairly standard, as treatment facilities often partnered with a place that did some kind of secondary housing, and you would get a job in the treatment facility. So you'd be living there, getting yourself together, with hope for a future. It's different now. Insurance and the healthcare industry doesn't want to foot the bill. You get a couple weeks, and then you're sent back out. Many people have complex medical, mental and physical health issues; it's not enough time. So someone using drugs who wants to make a change in their life feels stuck. They go, "Why bother even checking myself in. [These centers] don't offer what I need. There's not enough time, not enough beds." Never mind getting people treated by medical professionals prescribing safer medications. Forget buprenorphine or methadone or medical cannabis or anything. They never get to that point. They think, "I already tried that, and they kicked me to the streets."

The treatment industry is unique, in the sense it's the only one with a 7% success rate, but they blame the clients!

Not that it's all gloom and doom. I think many [in the recovery community] have learned we need to change and grow to meet an increasingly diverse clientele. One size *doesn't* fit all. Someone who uses only stimulants, for instance, needs a different plan and approach than another who uses strictly opiates. When I first started going to meetings, you'd have these old-timers who'd say that people on psych meds were not sober. That was like a very common attitude. That isn't the norm anymore, as people have grown more accepting that some may need medication. That's what so much of illicit drug use is, self-medication. Isn't it better to have your doctors, working with each other, come up with a treatment plan? And if that involves psyche meds or suboxone, that's better than someone going to a meeting and feeling they have to lie. It's certainly better than watching people you care about stop taking their doctor's advice, relapse, and die.

For me, harm reduction and 12 Steps programs are not at odds with each other. It's the people in the meetings that make the environment feel welcoming and supportive. That was the original idea for AA: a mutually supportive society. And we got away from that in some ways. In the original text of the Big Book, they talked about controlling drinking, they addressed going out and trying to control drinking—which is moderation management. I think, in some ways, they had a better handle on certain aspects of dependency in the '30s, because along the way members started making addendums and additions, where the approach got away from addressing problems using drugs and/or alcohol. You had people writing pamphlets and trying to control people's lives by saying, "You can only make it *one* way—*my* way." How is that helpful? People naturally resist being told how to live their lives, and even if you're trying to get them to a better place, they might not be able to see or hear—or appreciate—that if you come at them from such a dodged, stolid perspective.

Another factor that led me to harm reduction is more personal. My father died from alcohol-related complications. He went to AA for five years and never got sober, but parts of his life *did* improve from his involvement with the program. My dad liked the social element of the meetings. Attending them helped reduce his drinking and allowed him to enjoy a quality of life he didn't have previously.

I grew up in the Midwest. These days, it seems like everyone is addicted to opiates, which has forced certain issues into the open. Back then? People didn't talk about this stuff.

My mother died four months after my father. Her whole life's work was taking care of him and his alcoholism. My mom started going to Al Anon in the '70s. Back then, it was all tough love. My sister had a drug problem. They told her lock her out of the house. This was standard practice and advice for parents. We're talking the Scared Straight-era, Care Unit Incorporated, whose philosophy was, if your child is using drugs and tries to come home high, put a lock on the door, shut them out in the cold, get them to rehab, and call the sheriff if don't consent or they leave. My mom didn't believe in any of that shit. There was a lot of peer pressure for her to believe in it. And when I was very deep in my own addiction, she experienced significant social stigma. My mom went to 12 Step and Al Anon meetings to try to get a handle on her family's issues, to try and better understand, so she could help. She couldn't take that advice to turn your back on the people you loved. That was her firm belief: you had to love the person. That's amazing. Even if you didn't agree with them. For my mother, love was free, and it's the cornerstone of the relationship you want to have, even if the rest of that foundation is crumbling. She didn't believe withholding love, for whatever reason, was a good strategy.

When I went home in 1994, I told her the truth. I said, "I'm a bisexual junky prostitute. And if you can't accept me, I'm going to jump on the first freight train and turn around." And she said, "Well, I think you need some rest." That meant so much to me— that feeling of safety and care. She's the one who took me to get my AIDS test when they thought I had AIDS. Turned out, I had thrush really bad. But she didn't know that! My mom took me in her old Buick to get a to get an AIDS test. That's who she was. You just don't cut people off. She could've, and people would have understood. She dealt with my dad. She's already had gone through this with my sister. But she never let those experiences jade her or let it turn her heart to stone.

So all of my family, except for my mother, have had issues with drug or alcohol. And most of us have faced serious consequences from them.

I had thirty-four abscesses. I had Hep A, B and C, which I got rid of. I have problems with my teeth, which I mostly got fixed. I have vascular problems in my feet.

I consider myself lucky I haven't had worse health problems. And it's not like it's getting better out there.

I get so frustrated with some of the discussions around San Francisco because nobody wants to live in those unsafe, unclean conditions. You need access to sterile water and clean syringes. When you're out on the street, you have so much to contend with—street violence and rape, despair and infections. Then I'll hear, "Oh, that person's treatment resistant." Infuriating! These people are hurting, they *want* to change, but sometimes they can't meet that help where it's coming from. They're not in the right space. They can be dealing with psychiatric and mental health issues. Add drugs to the mix? Only compounds the problem. And if you're a member of a marginalized community—lesbian, gay, youth runaways, trans people—it only gets tougher. Those of us in recovery need to offer a safe haven.

I lived in an SRO (single room occupancy) hotel for sober living, which was run by the Salvation Army, for four years back when I was putting my life back together—so the mid-'90s. These rooms are disgusting. Even the "nicer" ones are disgusting. You live in a box; the room is like the size of a jail cell, and the things that I've seen in some of those hotels... I had a friend who was raped trying to go the bathroom. She was just walking down the hall to try to get the bathroom. The social isolation of living in some of those places will drive people to drugs and mental illness.

When I stayed in those hotels, you would really see the lack of hope. To bring it back to harm reduction, we're in a very dangerous time: the fentanyl era. There's a new level of urgency. You used to be able to hold off on stuff like that. I don't feel like you can hold off it on anymore. I work with parents. And I tell these parents, I think you should go find your child and try to talk to them and build a rapport. I'm not saying that you pull them off the street, but what I'm saying is take them out to lunch, go to the Tenderloin. Say you want to get lunch, and you use the time to work on a relationship. You don't have talk about their drug use at all. Go out to lunch with them. Go to a movie. You don't need to discuss what you both already know. They're on drugs, right? Go have these conversations with them where you tell them that you love them. I always tell the parents, you don't have to have them living at your house. You don't have to give them money. They'll understand why you're not giving them money, but there's other things you can offer. Let them know they are loved. Because that might be what helps them today. And you don't know when—or if—you'll get another chance.

Tracey can be reached at traceyh415@gmail.com

KYLE JOHNSTON

Lately, I've found some people on the social app Tik-Tok, who, like me, have transitioned from 12 Steps programs to harm reduction models. Turns out, many of us have similar upbringings. We do okay with the 12 Steps. Until we start speaking out against the harms and injustices that happen inside a 12 Step space, shortly after being ostracized; we need a little more support and encouragement than what AA offers.

My brothers and I were raised by a single mom, who I found dying suddenly when I was eleven. There were no hugs, words of support—just a funeral. There was no chance at closure.

We were sent to live with our mother's brother. We didn't know him that well. One of the first nights we were staying with him, he pulled us out of our beds at two in the morning. He sat us down in the living room, and said to us, "You're not going to kill me like you killed your mother." That was the beginning of the end of my youth and happiness. As if losing my mom wasn't enough, now we got Michael Jackson's father in charge.

Our uncle was responsible for raising us now, and he taught us the way he was taught. He was very old school in his views of what it meant to be a man. Hard knocks, I guess you could say. Literally. My brother and I learned how not to stand next to each other. Because if our uncle's mad, he'll take our heads and smack them together. He did that a lot. If my uncle didn't like what one of us had to say, he would smack us upside the head, leaving our ears ringing. This was the household I grew up in. When I got older and big enough to defend myself, I still wasn't ready to leave. As a victim of trauma, you grow used to the abuse. That's how it was with my uncle. I'd grown used to feeling that anxiety of him coming home and searching out these failures. Then one day, I got tired of getting beaten up. I looked at him and I said, "You're not going to touch me anymore." So he took all my stuff, and I ended up walking out of there with whatever I could carry in black bags. And this is the beginning of me finding people that would support me.

I ended up couch-surfing a lot. I ended up living with strangers. I've had moments where I've slept on park benches next to bus stops. So I can jump on the bus in the daytime. I also remember those moments random people would show me true human compassion.

I slept at this one bus stop for three days. I kept noticing this girl who was around my age. I must've been fifteen, sixteen at the time. After a few days of me going back to sleep at the bus stop, this girl comes over, looks at me, and says, "Follow me." I'm hungry. I'm cold. I followed her. She takes me to her family's house. When I walk in, there's a mother, father and three other kids. They asked if I needed a place to stay. I was allowed to live in that house for a year! Which is amazing. But I was hurting inside. And I never paid attention to that. I just went wherever it felt comfortable.

When I fell into drug addiction—well, before that I was a Marine. Which is a strange pathway to serving one's country. But I landed in the Marines because one summer I met a girl who told me I was cute. We dated all summer. Then one day she says, "I'm going to the Air Force." I figured it was one of those flings. But when she came back from boot camp, she found me and said, "Let's start a family." My decision-making wasn't at its best. She became pregnant. At this point, I'm living in my aunt's house, sleeping in the closet. I spent my days in the closet because she didn't want people to know I was there. I couldn't sleep on the couch, or in one of her spare beds. I was literally sleeping in a closet at the age of twenty-three. I had a child on the way. It was at this point, I told myself I need to go do something. Make something of myself so I can be a good father. I wanted to be the father I'd never had. So I joined the Marines. Shortly after boot camp, I received the Dear John letter. She wrote, "I don't need you anymore. You can go live your life." My motivation for the Marine Corps is gone. I gave up and began to drink heavily—which wasn't much of a leap. I was a Marine! I already drank like one. I prided myself on being the best drinker.

When I got my wisdom teeth pulled out, medics gave me my first prescription of Percocet. We called these med centers "Percocet tents." I became known around that base as the guy to go to for drugs. At that time, I didn't know how precious the drugs were. They continued to fill my script for my pain in my mouth for about four months. Then they stopped giving me the pills. No one prepared me for what came next.

Leaving the military, I'm out of meds. I'm on a Greyhound bus back to Ohio. And I start withdrawing. Once I get to Ohio, I'm sick. I talked to a friend, I tell them, "Man, I think I got the flu on the Greyhound!" He says, "You don't have a fever. You don't have the flu—you're dope sick."

This is where I learned about a world of pills and other things that would make me feel better. Military living had left me sheltered. As a Marine, I was in a constant state of fight-or-flight. But now, left alone with my own thoughts, I started dealing with all those emotions I'd suppressed—depression, anxiety, and fear. I was filled with a pervasive sense of impending doom, like something horrible would happen any moment. I ended up getting mixed up with a guy that sold drugs. Heroin. And while he sold heroin, I was the odd, weird black kid. I watched anime. I played video games. I listened to the Bee Gees. One day, he asked me to help sell those drugs. And I went from selling them to doing them. It seems crazy, but I was expected not to be doing them. Like that was a rule. We sold, we didn't use. Of course, I couldn't do that.

One day he asked me, point blank, "Are you on this shit?" And I was like, No! Why would you say that? He said, "Because you're walking around the house with your eyes closed." I acted offended. I said, "No! I would never do heroin."

In my mind, I wasn't like these other people we sold to. I was chipping, skimming off the top. I wasn't aware of how bad it was. This was how I spent my mid- to late-twenties and into my thirties. I battled. Not just with heroin—I battled with keeping up the ruse. I battled with getting up every day. I battled with the going out boosting, lying, stealing to get what I needed, finding people who had what I needed, and taking it from them, one way or another.

I got together with, what in AA they call "a hostage." This was a woman I became involved with, a partner, who had three kids. And soon the police would be involved. I was staying at what they call a trap-house—basically a crack house. And she showed up because I had been gone from home for three days. And she looks at me and the kids are in the car crying because they want me back. I wasn't worried about that. Because I'd turned into this very unpleasant person. I was doing them a favor not being around. She looks at me and says, "Kyle, I'm pregnant." And I said, "No, you're not. You're lying. You're just saying that because you want to get me home." I was like, "I can't come home because all you do is yell at me and you don't help me. But she also was addicted to heroin because of me." She'd had a car accident that shattered her ankle and required seven surgeries. She knew I was on Percocet. She didn't know I was on heroin. Every once in a while, she would ask me for a Percocet, to help with the pain and to relax. I always crushed it up for her. And one day I didn't have Percocet. I had heroin.

Eventually, I returned home. Then I went out boosting with a guy. I come back, go upstairs to shoot up. I'm an IV user at this point. I was one of the best. I got the biggest veins in the world. I never missed! Then I hear in the hallway. "Mr. Johnston, it's over! Come out with your hands up." The kids are like, "The cops are outside the door." I'm like, "Why'd you let them in?" The police handcuffed me and walked me out the house for the last time. I did not care about the kids. I did not care about the girl. I cared about the drugs upstairs that I just got and now won't be able to use. That's what I'd become.

I ended up in Cleveland, Ohio, county jail. They'll rank these things. Out of the "Ten Worst Jails To Be In America," Cuyahoga County has four. It was bad. I spent five months there. I detoxed in there. When the judge learned I was a veteran, I was placed in the Veterans' Drug Treatment Court. During my arraignment, they told me I was being sent to Stella Maris. Stella Maris is a behavioral health treatment center, which is where they let the clients—the residents— run the community. It's a hardcore but therapeutic community. It was my first time in treatment. Stella Maris was big on rules. But the biggest ones: read the Big Book, get a sponsor, stay out of trouble. I was there for six months. I got sponsors. I got a lot of them. And I kept getting different ones because I didn't like being told what to do or how to do it.

We're sitting there in the community room, and this guy comes in. One of the AA big shots. He's beating his chest, all tough. "I got twenty-eight years in this program, and I'm gonna show you how to keep it!" And he takes my hand, looks at me, and says, "Repeat after me." I nod. "He goes, You got a kid." I said, "Yeah." He said, "What you got." I said, "I got a girl." He says, "Okay. So, say fuck your daughter." And I try to pull my hand away. He don't let go. I tell him, "No, I'm not saying that!" He's like, "Say it. That's what you was saying when you was getting high." They use these narratives to scare you, belittle you, strip away your humanity.

I was forced to say, "Fuck my daughter," for him to let go of me. Yeah. But it was a lie. Just because I was using drugs didn't mean I didn't care about my daughter. But that's the narrative in that fellowship. Like, if you're getting high, you don't care about your family. That's not true. I had made some mistakes—some very big ones. But that didn't render me incapable of loving my kid.

I did six months there at a time, and I left. I had my daughter, I'm sitting at home, I'm starting to use heroin again. I started using Suboxone, but I wasn't using it right. And I was looking at her crawl on the floor. And as I'm watching her crawl, in my mind, I'm like, I should feel better about watching her grow up. Then when she started walking I'm, like, I should be proud that she's walking, but I couldn't appreciate that, because I was miserable with how I was living.

The only thing I ever heard about recovery was AA. So I called and went back to Stella Maris. Only this time, I'm working the program. But I'm making changes to it. I'm working it my way. Yeah, it's a lot of AA. It's a lot of other things too. I started adopting harm reduction. I knew some of these people might not totally stop. That didn't mean they didn't deserve help.

I'd watch people of all walks of life come in there, through all those things that you go through when you're sitting in a detox room without what you're used to. I didn't agree with that. I didn't view recovery as requiring punishment first.

I began adopting this philosophy into how I treated and helped others. People would come to Stella Maris detox because they'd say they knew Kyle's gonna be there. And I'm gonna be treated fairly, because not everybody is treated right in recovery. We all know about the health care system in America and how treatment centers are really focused on that money.

When I left detox that first time, I wasn't ready. I was now. By this time, I am like four years into it. I've created my own meetings, ones that that didn't just say "AA or bust!" I started to bring in outside information. Many of the old-timers shunned me for that. They said I was headed for a relapse if I read anything other than the Big Book. They'd see me with new reading material and ask, "What book is that?!" And I'd say, "Oh, it's a smart recovery book." And they'd be, all, "Burn it!" Like this was the 1600s and I was practicing witchcraft.

So I had to move on. I ended up working for a place called Thrive Behavioral Health, where I became a care coordinator. As a case manager, I oversaw people who wanted peer support. This was my introduction to peer support. I had a caseload of 275 clients. Holy shit! Which I'm pretty sure isn't even legal.

That was the demand, though. We all had a very seriously high caseload. And we did treatment plans, intakes, Bio/psycho/socials, we did crisis calls. That was the first time I had a crisis call where a young lady was talking about killing herself. And I was talking to her, reasoning with her. I'm waving my hands in the air to get someone's attention. I'm telling them to call the police as I'm keeping her on the phone. And fifteen minutes later, she's like, "Kyle, fuck you!" And the cops are like come on then and then I find out three months later that she's in treatment and she's happy to be there.

But this is the moment where my life was impacted to the point where I had changed gears. While working at Thrive, I met someone named Ashley Rosser. She's not just gorgeous; she is like a real human being. She does harm reduction. She does outreach. She will go out and set up tables and pass out Narcan, give out information about substance use, and tell people about stigma. When I met her, I was this really loving guy, but I had had a 12 Step stigmatized brain chip put in my head. We'd talk about recovery, but like not recovery as I'd been taught. She would tell me about living and harm reduction.

Then I'm back at work, and I'm sitting there and I'm listening to all these clients with these stories about how they had been mistreated by their sponsor, how this person took advantage of them. This person started messing with their wife, this person fought them, and then there was a rape here and like all these crimes, like truly by the book. I'm looking at my superiors, asking, "What do we do?" And they're like, "Well, that's not our problem." I'm still going to meetings, but now I'm starting to speak up. When I hear somebody badgering or belittling somebody, I'm like, "Where does it tell you to do that in the Big Book?" Where does it tell your sponsee not to read the book by themselves? Where in the book does it stipulate a newcomer can't talk for a year. Somebody, please show me where it says that. And I get people looking at me, like, now I'm a problem. Why? Because I'm challenging them. These old schoolers. I'm challenging how they've always done things. But sometimes the way you're doing things can work in some ways, while other parts can be broken. I've been to the sober houses that are little more than squats. They have roaches and infestations and leaky walls and busted beds. But it's still a three-bedroom house with twelve people crammed in, each paying four, five, six hundred bucks to live in the shithole. And then they're told to be grateful!

After talking to Ashley, I got shaken up. I said, "Hey, guys, we can do better." We can be more loving. We can actually do what the Big Book says. Then I challenged them too much. I said the information in the book—which was written a hundred years ago—doesn't always coincide with what science and evidence-based knowledge tells us today. We're truly harming people and setting them up for a premature failure. And they looked at me, and they laughed at me. Then they shamed me. Yeah. So I went home. And at this time, I was in a relationship. I looked at my partner at the time, and I said, "I want to do something different." And she's like, "What do you mean?" And I said, "I want to stand up. And I want to say out loud: this needs to stop." And she told me she was with me, and believed in me. And when I told her I wouldn't be able to keep my job, she said, "Well, you can put in your two weeks' notice." This is where Drop the Label started.

Drop the Label was an idea that came around because as I was learning about harm reduction. I started learning the definitions of mental health and substance misuse. I started reading books and listening to seminars that spoke about the negatives words, and the stigma they carry. And I'm like, "Wow! Everything we say in AA stigmatizes." Like, we're walking around going, "Hey, I'm an addict. I can never be cured or normal." That's stigmatizing.

The first 164 pages of AA's Big Book has never been revised. Society has changed, the world is different—they've made additions to the stories section—but that part, the hallmark of AA, has never been amended. Not one iota. The idea that once an addict, always an addict is paralyzing. Just because you were in addiction doesn't mean you're always going to be one. Rejecting that doesn't afford the possibility of change. It keeps you chained. Because no matter how far you go, that disease is always going to be there. Through harm reduction, I've come to view this condition of drug use and misuse as a spectrum.

I started Drop the Label because you'd have newcomers showing up to meetings and being told to stop taking their psyche meds. Taking mental health meds won't kill you. But not taking them just might. Still, you'd get these old-timers telling people who were sick beyond excessive alcohol or drug use that as long as they were taking physician prescribed medication, "You're not sober." It's just so hypocritical. The first line of the Big Book dictates that no 12 Step staff member is a doctor and to leave medication to the professionals! But most of them don't listen.

This didn't make me popular in the traditional recovery community. As I'm doing this, I'm losing friends—I'm losing places that I can go where I'm comfortable. As I'm doing this, I am being ostracized. Every day, I'm coming home with this pain of loss. And I really didn't think that these people that I had been walking with for four years, that know my heart—that showed up to my birthdays, and my surprise anniversaries of my sobriety date—I never thought these people I considered friends would not be here for me. I had one sponsee, who was living in a sober house, call me in the middle of the night, saying he was either smoking crack or killing himself. He was getting harassed that bad. How is that recovery?

This is why I started Drop the Label, and it's why I continue it to this day. Drop the Label represents compassion, speaking out loud for what you need for you to succeed. And the message has resonated. I've been flown out to speak in places like Chicago. I am seated next to authors of books that have gotten big awards, next to White House officials sitting with their doctors—big names in the recovery community—and there's people in the audience there to hear me speak.

Drop the Label has helped pave a new path to recovery. Through it, I get to talk about harm reduction and stigma. I get to pass out harm reduction literature. I get to find people that are living in tents, and you know, in the woods or under the bridge, and offer them services, give them food, clothing, hygiene, get them into our shelter. Or if we don't have space, we're going to pay for a week at a hotel. We want people feeling comfortable with who they are again.

When people like this can relax, they travel back in time, see a world of possibility and hope. Sometimes, they slip up. That's okay. We'll try again. When people slip in AA, it fast turns into a relapse, and they crumble because they are never taught how to stand up on their own. Drop the Label is about getting people back on their own two feet and helping them stay there. And if they stumble from time to time? We're there to offer a little support until they're feeling steady again and they can stand on their own again. We aren't there to shun or shame. Drop the Label is community designed to encourage and empower.

Kyle can be reached at Kjaveragejoe@gmail.com

AZZY-MAE NI MHAILLE

My story starts before I entered public health. I developed a fascination with mind alteration and substance consumption at a very early age. I experimented with various substances, and was pretty methodical in how I did it. I was lucky enough to be on a drug checking seminar recently. I got to hear from the creators of Erowid. It was amazing to be around two people—even virtually—who had such a profound effect on my life. And two people, without whom, I wouldn't be engaging in this level of harm reduction.

When I was using, there was all sorts of different genres of consumption. Some were more, I guess, eclectic. The more focused consumption happened in my twenties. A best friend of mine at the time and I used to talk about the experience, the subtle nuances between different types of drug use. And I'd say my introduction to harm reduction was the result of mindful consumption—this idea of "risk reduction" that we were practicing.

I engaged in the illicit substance trade for a good period of time. And during that time I'd be working with people who I was distributing to—to make sure that they were educated on the substances that they were going to take. And often what that looked like was me having consumed the substance first. This way I could give them both an objective and a subjective analysis. I had to the point where it would be like, "Hey, are you taking any medications?" And "if you're taking X, Y, and Z medication, this substance isn't for you." Which *is* harm reduction.

My career in public health began the summer of 2016. In my hometown, a syringe had washed up on one of the beaches. And a child stepped on it. There was a public uproar. This was shortly after my late best friend had passed away. My uncle had also passed away. *Both* from overdoses. Within a week of my uncle's passing, I was on Facebook. My hometown board was discussing this incident on the beach. At this time, I was completely abstinent from substances and engaging in the 12 Step fellowship. I was also actively working to destigmatize drug use. So when there was this post, *a lot* of people were outraged, which left me with no choice but to say that approach was unhelpful. I mean, the things being said about people who used drugs – we didn't even know if this needle that washed up was related to substance consumption. But I was engaged in a comment section (people aren't human on Facebook or in comment sections) and this woman is just spewing a lot of drug-use stigma. I spewed right back, like, "Hey, that's, you know, mean and unproductive! What we really need to be doing is focusing on support options and proper disposal." This woman said something—I'll never forget it. She said, "If you're such a wealth of information, I guess we'll see you at the town hall tomorrow!" I took it as a challenge. Well, all right, I guess you will!

The following day was the service for my late uncle. I went directly from the service, still dressed in my Sunday best—and this was, y' know, pre-transition. So I was all suited up. And I stood up at that city hall meeting, with people talking big, about how, "If we see somebody on the beach who looks like they're consuming substances, we should pull out our camera phones!" Others were clamoring how there should be cameras installed on the beach. It was a lot of really outlandish, non-helpful ideas. I got up the nerve to get up and speak. I talked about my experience with it. I didn't hold back. I talked about needles and injection—intravenous drug consumption. I also pointed out how ridiculous it was that people would be shooting up on a beach. If you've ever been on the coast, you know how heavy the winds get. Makes prep impossible. Plus, sand gets everywhere.

Afterwards, my former executive director came up to me and said, "Hey, we're looking to start a syringe exchange locally, and we'd like you to be involved in that." It had been a while for me. I considered my career to be in the restaurant industry. I'd worked in the field from thirteen to twenty-five. But I was tired of it. I didn't feel like I wanted to continue in that industry. The late nights, the even later mornings—they weren't vibing with what I envisioned for my life. And just as I'm thinking of making a change, I'm presented with this opportunity. And this felt more like *me*. I get to go out and offer support to people I really cared about? Get access to treatment and care? Yes! This was the logical next step. And that's what began (what will soon be) a seven-year career in public health, with a focus on a more formalized from of harm reduction.

With the opening of the syringe access program, I hit the ground running. This experience in needle exchange is how I got to meet my harm reduction heroes, Eliza Wheeler, Gary Langis, Sarah Mack, and Megan Hines. It was truly a trip to meet these people who are doing such amazing work, and so early on in the game! It helped to have such strong role models within the field. They set a powerful example for me.

We started by doing mostly syringe access but that soon expanded to overdose education and naloxone distribution through the Pilot Project in Massachusetts. So I'd be doing Narcan trainings for that organization as well. And then at work, doing Hep C, HIV, STD testing, a lot of street outreach at that first spot, and then also speaking, either through Act Up or on an independent basis to various schools and organizations, which all centered around ideas around harm reduction. This was my entry into consulting as well.

I now work out of Boston, where I've done a lot of street out-reach, as well as some drop in-style interventions. In the past year, I've been managing a navigation center for women and trans folks, cis women and trans folks, rather—people who either are experiencing homelessness, or who are engaging in sex work and who consume substances. Really, anyone who wants to join the program.

Coming from a 12 Step experience, where there's this culture of silence around risk reduction conversations. There's this implied threat with AA, how if you engage in behavior they don't condone, you'll be exiled from that program—people will be told not to associate with you, because now you're one of the losers.

In addition to that, I've been working with things like risk reduction, which is one of my favorite groups. Risk Reduction groups are the reason I jaywalk significantly less now. Because we would always have to give an example of a risky behavior we'd like to address, and I wouldn't want to necessarily center my lived experience in those conversations. Jaywalking was a risky behavior I felt comfortable talking about. I'd say, "Well, it gets me there quicker." But there's the risk of getting struck by a car. So we talked about that. What could I do to help reduce risk? Well, I take my headphones off, then I look both ways. And those are two risk reduction steps that I can take that aren't abstinence, but they could, potentially, save my life.

Hegemonic control over discourse, and action that is maintained by abstinence only, is really tying the hands of what could be extremely effective and holistic programs that recognize what a varying population needs.

I think a lot of this comes from the monetization of the practice. When we talk about these [12 Step groups] despite criticism, we also recognize that some people have benefited from them. It's a question of changing culture. Personally, I didn't *really* start to grow until I felt confident within my own harm reduction practices. This has involved attempts at moderation. Through trial and error, I was able to find things that worked for me.

I remember the meeting where I made my decision to leave 12 Steps. I was the secretary of my home group. I can't remember who the bookie was but they brought in any yeller. This guy got up in front of the room and was yelling his share. And this man had the nerve to sit in front of a room of people and say, "Yeah, I Thirteen Step. I'm sick. That's why I'm here."

I checked out immediately. That was the moment where I was,

like, Listen, I can appreciate if you're working in a program of abstinence from substances, and that you are actively working on who you are as a person. More power to you. But if you are abstinent from substances, and you are not working on yourself, you are leveraging power dynamics within the community—you're harming people. I just don't see the utility there.

I saw a culture of misogyny within AA—a culture of science denial. There was this universal shutdown of any other potentially helpful behavioral health methods. It has turned into a culture of really putting down anyone who wasn't doing things the *exact* way that was prescribed by some home group or sponsor.

I just flat out rejected it. I need to do things that are going to keep me safe. *I* get to decide that. So I walked away from that culture of ignoring—ignoring the material conditions that inform problematic relationships to substances. Like, disease model essentialism that ignores everything else that plays out outside of the person.

I believe that harm reduction is the pursuit of health wellness and risk reduction from everyday behaviors. And I think that it could look like anything from taking off your headphones when you're trying to cross the street, to going to a drug checking site to make sure that the substance that you're about to consume is the substance that you're looking to be consuming, all the way to participating in a treatment for problematic relationships to substances. So long as that is a *voluntary* action and not being coerced. I think any of those things could be harm reduction.

I truly believe that the essence of harm reduction is any positive change—any steps taken to improve one's health and wellness and reduce risk. And I don't see a definition of that word that doesn't include science-backed treatment. I believe abstinence-only based programs enforce a culture upon people, people who are not necessarily voluntarily consenting to it. I don't view that as something that's harm reducing. I think that if somebody wants to volunteer themselves for treatment, excellent. I think forcing people into treatment flies in the face of harm reduction. I think that it really boils down to the philosophy.

At its core, harm reduction is about mutual aid. People helping people to reduce potential dangers. And this can take all forms.

When it comes to the future of harm reduction, I'd like to see the United States catch up to what our neighbors up northing are doing, places like British Columbia, for sure. Globally, I would like to see harm reduction continue to pursue the decriminalization, if not legalization, of all substances. I'm fighting for liberation of mandatory treatment from this dominant discourse of abstinence-only. I'd like to see housing for all, and health care for all, because I think that those are among the biggest impediments within the US. I want us to share the amazing statistics we see out of countries that have those resources. I'm advocating for trans liberation and queer liberation. And let's tackle imperialism as well for that matter! *And* the chauvinistic nationalism that we have here within the US. I'd like to see harm reduction actively pursuing means to end chauvinism as well as to those overarching systems. Because I think that our climb is significantly steeper and significantly harder to navigate if those are impediments are there.

I think the one thing I would like people to understand about harm reduction is how far reaching it is in all contexts, but specifically how far reaching it is in the context of people who consume substances. How while it is extremely beneficial for people who have problematic relationships to substances, it is also beneficial to a wide range of people who don't have that experience with substance consumption and who still deserve all of the supports that we offer—all of the resources that we offer—because everybody deserves safety.

Azzy-Mae can be reached at Fratemaezrael@gmail.com

CHAD SABORA

For my harm reduction story, I need to go backwards, starting with my dad. My dad was in recovery and a pioneer in the field during his time. He found recovery in 1970, long before he met my mom. He was part of the first graduating class of Gateway Foundation, which then turned into an immediate hire because back in 1971 there were almost no official policies or practices for working in the field yet. My dad's story like many others, well, that's just how people went to work back then. And that led to Dad, with the rest of his graduating class, running Gateway House, which was rooted in all the old-school modalities we hear about today. Treatment back then was based on the principle of "building people up by first breaking them down." I mean, they would make people stand on a chair and scream to embarrass themselves. It was crazy! There's this movie Gateway put out, a documentary called "The Dwarf and the Giant" with my dad in it. It's surreal for me to watch. It's like watching *Shaft* because of the '70s style cinematography. Much like me, my dad was not ashamed or embarrassed to put his struggles out there for the public to see because he was a force of change in his own time. But dad was no longer working there and was instead an executive by the time I was able to understand things. And my mom was a prosecutor so we had incredible arguments at the dinner table, but always intellectually based conversations, often about drug use and the people who use them. I will admit, for a very long time, I tended to agree with my mom and I will also admit that I was wrong.

I was a bit reckless growing up. I pushed the limits of human existence wherever I could and that included my experimentation with drugs. However, I never had any problematic use whatsoever. I was one of those people that didn't understand why other people couldn't just stop. I was able to use for a weekend—go hit the West Side and grab some rocks and some China White [which] was called "blow" back in the 90s on the west side of Chicago. And when heroin first really hit the market here in 1993 – 94, I seriously couldn't get it, why other people couldn't stop. That ability I had was quickly taken away right after I graduated law school and I lost both of my parents to cancer eighteen months apart. My father passed away from leukemia in early 2005 and then in September of 2006 my mother passed away from numerous types of cancer, but I believe she actually died of a broken heart and the cancer just helped her get to where she wanted to be, which was with my dad. At that point I realized that when you are using drugs to self-medicate for another condition, mine being grief, you can no longer just put them down until the underlying issue has been resolved and healed. This time, I could not stop.

I have a psych background and a law degree, and an intelligence that makes me somewhat socially awkward. I found myself getting into harm reduction and drug policy reform because the system's broken. So, at the end of the day, I ended up working in this field and specifically in harm reduction following a "series of unfortunate events." Or maybe those events weren't unfortunate but a necessity for me to become who I was supposed to be. Getting into this work produced a profound change. I had truly found my passion, which is great, because I did *not* enjoy being an attorney. I honestly went to law school because I was bored and had no idea what I wanted to be when I grew up, and although I thoroughly enjoyed the education I received, the work was something that I really didn't give a shit about. There is one thing I know about myself and that is I was never meant to work at 9-to-5 job for somebody else for the rest of my life. To me that would be the equivalent of despair.

I remember in 2012 (I graduated high school in 1994) when I was first getting started in harm reduction, I had friends from high school who were dying from overdoses. By 2012 and 2013, I felt helpless watching them all die. But I also started thinking, "Here's something I can do with my white-ass privilege. Having that JD behind my name opens doors, so use it!" But I had also been indoctrinated to the 12 Steps and seeing all that bullshit, and breaking away from it, it's almost like getting deprogrammed and suddenly being able to see the bigger picture. At one point I really wanted to do this massive campaign, but nobody would give me the money. Sort of the equivalent of coming out of the closet. I wanted to get people who work in the field to admit to their past discriminatory beliefs towards drug use, towards recovery. And I wanted to get them to say, "This was my aha moment," and get a lot of people with big names, a bunch of others, maybe even some celebs, to "come out." Basically, I wanted to give people the space to be vulnerable. Why? Because I can't isolate my "aha moment." I just discovered the most effective way to save lives is harm reduction and I jumped right into it.

I'm also very rebellious by nature so I was more than happy to break the law when it came to naloxone distribution and putting my neck out there in a calculated way, because I had already secured my immunity from arrest and other things. But, you know, I learned that I have the ability to navigate the political and socioeconomic system of the country and make positive change. I was lucky to get into this field when Dan Bigg and others were still with us. Unfortunately, Edith Springer had already passed. There were so many of the original people still around when I got into harm reduction that I was able to be tutored—and (I say lovingly) in a very abusive way by Dan Bigg! Now I look at these kids coming into the work and I want to say to them, "You have no idea *who* your history is." So not only did I find passion, I also found a responsibility, like the one that was given to me that I didn't want—the responsibility to teach these youngsters about our collective harm reduction history. I remember in 2019 a bunch of us were brought to Nashville. The guest list was organized by Daniel Raymond and Tom Hill, I think it was the NatCom conference? Me, Jess Tilly, Mark Jenkins, Jesse Harvey, Chase Hollerman, Jenna Sheldon. Lots of people. And in retrospect, I can see what that meeting was for. They picked us for future leadership. Shortly after that conference, a few people that I considered some of my closest friends and allies died and then Daniel Raymond left the field as did Kiefer, Paterson, and others. Leaders like Eliza Wheeler had moved into different areas and we all felt like there was this void left. None of us felt we had the ability to fill those shoes. And I think we're still kind of fumbling with leadership a bit. I know I have the knowledge to debate— and I do that a lot in social media, and in my writing and my videos—but it's like that role that Dan Bigg had, that Mark Kinzly had … I don't know if there's another giant out there. That's why I got involved in harm reduction and that's why I stayed, because somebody has to teach harm reduction the right way to the next generation.

Even in the leadership area, there're people I have issues with when it comes to understanding what harm reduction really is. Harm reduction is a byproduct of social justice reform and understanding equity and systemic racism and basically the structure of America. The fact that I got into massive, systemic, federal drug policy reform and harm reduction just happened to be an area that I also got good at, and my past experience as a drug user became really, really helpful. But my entry point into harm reduction was broader than just alcohol and other drugs, and the breadth of my work that I now try to focus on, it's definitely more than drug harm reduction. But harm reduction falls under the bigger "social justice" umbrella. That's why I stay. I'm not really sure where our leaders are on some issues. But I sure don't want to be one of those leaders even though I've been made a quasi-leader. It's an unwilling appointment for sure!

All of this is to say that harm reduction to me is very different than what it means to a lot of others, including other harm reductionists. It's also hard to define. In its simplest form, just flip the words: it's *reducing harm*. It's also an attempt to mitigate the damages caused by human nature and our needs because it goes beyond drug use. For instance, the other authors of the federal harm reduction framework and I, all met in Rockville, MD, in the spring of 2024 to discuss the framework and to plan our next steps. It was brought up that sex workers got left out of the federal framework, which the Feds apologized for, but then they told us, "Well, we thought you would get enough comments submitted when the framework was released for the public." But they didn't tell us that! We managed to have a good conversation that day in spite of all that. Humans are beautiful, a beautiful species. I *want* to help them. I just don't want to talk to them most of the time. But at the same time, we have so *many* harms in our society, whether it be through drug policy, laws, systemic racism, xenophobia—and that list could go on and on. So, to me harm reduction is understanding that some of us need to take up the call to mitigate the harms that are caused by just being human beings. And that goes into a deeper understanding of sociology, human psychology, indoctrination, religious zealotry—so many things that make us so remarkably unique, and also make us the most dangerous mammals on the planet. There's so much harm caused by our nature as humans that can be mitigated by people who can find that balance and embody the line from the song "Imagine"—everyone living in peace. There are people out there—I consider myself one of them—including people I work with, where we can be both at peace and in chaos. That meme of the dog drinking coffee in a house in flames saying, "Everything is okay?" That's my "comfy space." I'm happy in that space where you can see the world burning from people's actions, people's ignorance, people's awful ignorance, and from the lack of access to education. The harm reduction I do seeks to absolve that, even though I also know that's never going to go away completely. But we can reduce the harms we know are a natural consequence of the human journey. This is *my* view of harm reduction.

Harm reduction is such a complicated thing to define because it's *not* what people think it is. I would challenge people to seek a definition that goes beyond recovery and goes beyond the use of drugs. I would continue to let them grapple with what they think I want to hear. I don't want to give people *the answer.* I want to let them know that 98.5% of them are wrong, and that they need to conceptualize things outside the moral framework that we currently possess, and give me a better answer, and a better understanding of what harm reduction means. I would say, "Recognize your own misconceptions, if you have the courage to be open minded, and do your due diligence, because there's so many misconceptions about harm reduction." So many people have titles such as "Harm Reduction Training Specialist" in their email signatures. Really? You took a course from somebody who doesn't even know what they're talking about and now you're calling yourself a harm reductionist? Recently somebody said that Robert Ashford, a researcher I work with, is not a harm reductionist. "What?" I want to say to them, "You mean he's not a harm reductionist the way *you* think he should be, which is 'boots on the ground?'" But that's not what defines a harm reductionist. What defines harm reduction is how we see the world. Because Robert is 100% a harm reductionist—his research—everything. The fact that he doesn't do direct services or such doesn't mean shit.

Another example of what I'm talking about was when the harm reduction community lost one of its most loved members and somebody who I considered one of my closest friends, Dean Lemire. Dean was an amazing and beautiful human being. A few months before his passing, he and I had launched a national harm reduction education program that truly could have changed things for so many. A few days after he passed away another guy in Missouri, who does harm reduction training, made a comment to me that, "I hope his death doesn't reflect negatively on the harm reduction community." I had to say to him, "And that comment is why you're not a harm reductionist. If your immediate concern is how the community will possibly be harmed by Dean's death, you're a *recovery* person, not a harm reduction person." Coming from a harm reduction perspective, Dean's passing was tragic, and involved so many personal struggles and demons that at the end of the day, he was just another victim of our war on drugs who was working on the front lines. And that's the risk many of us take in this field. His death would have no impact on our harm reduction community because we understand the value of human life and the value of living experience. He doesn't get that we harm reductionists are the agents of change *and* we're also a lot of the casualties. That's what a harm reductionist would look at when they see Dean's death. What this guy saw was some 12 Step or church-based version where he's concerned Dean's death will have a negative impact on the harm reduction community. We don't give a shit, and that's the difference between him and us. I say all this because Dean was one of my best friends. I can look to situations like that and say Robert Ashford is absolutely a harm reductionist because of his philosophical belief system about how he sees the world. And if you can't grasp that, no matter what you're doing on the streets, maybe *you're* the one who's not a harm reductionist!

Part of the problem today is if you're not passing out syringes you're not seen as a harm reductionist. I did that work for ten years. But I'm better at policy work. I want to say these folks that the reason why you have naloxone to pass out is because

I'm behind the computer all day working to pass laws on naloxone, and other people are writing books, and we do things to make the use of naloxone acceptable. There was a very understandable timeline from 1989 until today of people's actions that allow you "boots on the ground" folks to do what you do. So, I get frustrated with the fact that too many newer harm reduction folks don't understand their own history. That's why I take on some mentees and do the harm reduction history training. There are so many people that are some of the purest, most beautiful harm reductionists in the world and too many of these "kids" have never heard of them just because those harm reductionists aren't popular on social media or in the midst of the shit in Kensington. But that doesn't mean they're not harm reductionists.

I can just talk to a person and feel their energy and understand that this person does or does not see the world as a place where equity and access to care matters. You can also tell by who they vote for. Unfortunately, there is a political affiliation that comes with this work. And neither of the parties represent us—well, one of them kind of does. But if Kamala loses, we're screwed as far as harm reduction work goes. I live in a red state and I know too many people who lost someone who's in another red state but we've also lost some in blue states. I don't want to engage those who live in those red states most of the time. Dr. Katz actively blocked so much work we wanted to do that I wound up screaming at her on a public forum and I was asked not to return. But nobody, neither party talks about drugs. I heard someone say once we should put all the homeless people and drug addicts on an island. Wow. That is not harm reduction! There's just so many more things that are involved in this work than direct services to people who use drugs, and you can't embody everything that needs to be done, because nobody can. But there's people in those spaces that you owe respect to, like half of those kids don't know who Zach is, or Christopher who Zach does the podcast with. So, I keep saying to all of the players in harm reduction, "Sit down like I did and learn your history." I just wish people would be more intellectually curious instead of just, "I want to get popular and go do work." It's great that you want to do work, but first learn! I think this is a huge problem we're having right now with the younger generation—at least some of them.

I'm sure Dan said the same thing though ... and Edith and Dave Purchase. It's just that social media makes it a little more frustrating, especially when you look at efforts to end overdose and we see grant money getting taken by bad players out there and not going to the "boots on the ground" folks that have been doing that work forever. Harm reduction has a fiscal note attached to it now, which it never did and that brings out so many people that are career opportunists, pretending to do this work. And you know, if we don't stay diligent, we're going to be just phased out by these players and the system will take everything, so we have to be very proactive and have the courage to call people out. We have to stay true to what we've been given by those who came before us.

The only way I see change happening in both the policy area and in healthcare regarding harm reduction is to integrate it into the healthcare system. It already is for other conditions! I would like to see drug use and people with a substance use disorder to be recognized and identified as two distinct populations, and then let's see the health needs of those two populations be met by the primary health care system, where harm reduction already exists for other areas of health. Care would be in every building and area of healthcare where the capacity to treat those who want care for a substance use disorder could have it. This would just be part of our normal healthcare system where drug users could get better education on agonist therapy for instance and doctors would be better equipped on the unique considerations they need when dealing with somebody who uses drugs. Drug users should not have to go to a separate building, to other doctors, to get the care they want and need. This is the stigma that has to stop for things to really change. What does it matter if someone has a substance use disorder or they have a back problem? Let's just have everyone treated together in the same building, not another way a half mile down the road. That change would be real harm reduction to me and better policy all at once.

Chad can be reached at chad4harmredux@gmail.com

NJON SANDERS

There's a lot of misconception about what harm reduction is, which presents challenges in terms of navigating the recovery industry. Public figures and policy-makers don't understand what harm reduction entails, so when they raise objections, which on paper might seem like common sense; they get it wrong. However well-intentioned, those in charge of implementing policies help perpetuate these misconceptions. The solution is combining harm reduction with traditional methods of recovery, because those two aren't mutually exclusive.

Advocates of harm reduction aren't opposed to putting people in treatment—treatment often leads to positive outcomes—but the user needs to *want* that treatment; you can't force someone to *want* to get better. Mandated treatment seldom works. No one wants to be told what to do. Forcing treatment can, at times, be worse than *no* treatment. Often, the issue becomes political, further muddying already murky waters. When someone makes the *choice* to get help, they have a shot at success. Too many times, we see users—often younger users, from privileged, suburban backgrounds—who are mandated to get help, where they are placed in-patient and supervised, only to come out and overdose.

When I went to treatment, decades into my addiction (and after several failed attempts at sobriety), the facility offered medically assisted treatment, which I of course refused. Because I'd been conditioned to believe that "real recovery" meant no medications, no chemical assistance. Otherwise, it wasn't "real" sobriety. So I said, "No, thanks." In my mind, I needed to man up and go cold turkey. I'd been attending meetings for years and years, where people hammered this point, again and again. I'd hear, "You've been in these meetings for years. You need to listen to the way *we* tell you to do things. Stop being difficult and get with the program." At least, this is how I heard the messages.

And I kept coming up short, or in my mind I kept failing.

Luckily, I discovered LifeRing Secular Recovery, which supports multiple paths on the road to recovery. It's all about meeting people where they are. This approach led me to watching more media and reading more. Incorporating harm reduction with the LifeRing community was a no brainer. Many members of LR are people like me. They had been hammered with one-size-fits-all solutions—which is the total opposite of harm reduction.

When I later moved on to chair the San Francisco Behavioral Health Commission, I got to see firsthand a lot of the work that's currently being done in the harm reduction field, and how it affects real people, and how it impacts people's lives and helps transform them. By refuting the one-size punitive model, harm reduction has *shown* there is more than one way to fix a problem.

The key to wellness is "hope," which is a huge component to recovery. Without hope, how can an addict imagine getting better? By skipping this vital step, i.e., hope, many, including myself, were set up to fail. I've seen so many people who want to get better, and they are pushed to attend 12 Step meetings. There's a subtext that without meetings, you can't get better. Meetings can be great. But without first having that hope, recovery is not a realistic expectation.

I've been attempting recovery since the eighties. Back then, if you got into treatment, you were lucky. The only recovery option was 12 Step meetings. I was in Ohio. Sadly, there are still too many places where 12 Step is the default; it's ingrained, and the media popularizes it to this day. So as addicts, what do we do? We go to church basements, we cry, and we resign ourselves to hopelessness. We sit in a circle and talk about how our lives are terrible, and we're constantly on the brink of total disaster. What's missing? Hope!

I was at a conference a couple years ago, and there's a comedian that hits the recovery circuits. One of his jokes goes, "Oh, yeah, first thought, garbage." And it's like, no! Oftentimes, my instincts *are* correct. Oftentimes, my instincts protect me from a lot of harm. That's right. Sometimes when I'm afraid, or when something is intimidating to me, there's a good reason for it. Using might interfere with my strategy or means to an end, but that doesn't mean I shouldn't listen to myself. I don't necessarily need to do the *first* thing I think of, but it's certainly a good jumping off point.

Because not everything that we think as addicts is garbage or wrong. "My best thinking that got me here." Yeah. You know, it also got me out of that mess. And it's that duality, knowing the difference between good and "bad" thoughts. I must be able to visualize something that's not awful and terrible. What eventually got me back into recovery was just the hope of, "Okay, I can do this. I'm going to be miserable, because I was miserable in recovery previously, just by white-knuckling it, but that will be better than what I'm doing to myself using the way I am." The toll using was taking on my mental and physical health—it was too much. I was ready for *any* alternative, and I was shocked to find out that it didn't have to be awful. It didn't have to be on someone else's terms. This isn't to bash AA, but there *are* other ways out. I didn't have to be a follower, accepting that *everything* I thought was "stinkin' thinkin'." I have plenty of worthwhile ideas, using or not. This was liberating! I didn't have to listen to some schmuck who's been sober six months longer than I was tell me how to live my life. That kind of autonomy isn't encouraged in 12 Step. It's just not. Some people have no issues with that. But me? Yeah, I get to drive. I get to make the decisions. And positioning myself behind the wheel is how I got here, healthier and happier.

Recovery—especially in 1980's Ohio—felt like a competitive sport. Who could rack up the most sober time? Who gets to the finish line fastest? How many meetings did *you* get to in a week? Who has a more hardcore sponsor? Competition doesn't have to be bad, but in recovery, back then, I felt like this combative element was counterproductive. It was also ingrained in recovery culture back in the day. And unfortunately, I still see some of it lingering in a lot of the proselytizing [in our communities]. Turning recovery into a contest doesn't make a support group feel very supportive anymore.

I hate to see anyone struggle. It's hard for me to watch them struggle. At the end of the day, the solution is a simple one: branch off and do your own thing. If that's 12 Steps and meetings, great! If it's something like LifeRing, terrific! And if you have to carve your own unique niche? More power to you. I think users still have to make the choice, and be given the freedom to do what *they* believe is the path for *them*.

This harm reduction approach has impacted my professional life, as well. I started in general operations working for tech companies, kind of a jack of all trades, facilities and HR and IT, and now I specialize in People Operations. I'm a Senior People Partner at Elroy Air, where we're building a cargo drone for multiple uses in the humanitarian, military, and commercial sectors for carriers like FedEx to use between their distribution centers. I love my job. I love the people I work with. This all goes back to the volunteer work I've been doing over the past decade, which has gotten me to this point, where I'm coaching leaders, I'm coaching individual contributors and creating policies and processes that serve people; I help the company understand the value of taking care of its people. So we're working on our diversity, equity, inclusion, and belonging. This is a company-wide approach, tracking who we are and who we hire and who we choose to partner with—the kind of energy we want to put into our community and into the world. And it's been wonderful to have the freedom to do this. It's something I've been wanting to do for a very long time, and it took a while for me to build up the confidence, but a big part of my recovery journey has been the skills that I've learned by participating, speaking in meetings, and sharing my truth in public. I'll speak at conferences, volunteer on different boards and civic organizations, which has shown me how to get past the bullshit and get right to the heart of the matter, the meat: how do we best serve others?

And how do we do that? For me, it goes back to hope, and how are we demonstrating that you have options; there are ways that you can get to where you want, places that you hadn't previously been able to imagine for yourself. And we can help you get there. It's just a matter of doing the work—together. And we're going to support you. But *you* need to ask what *you* want. "Have you thought about X, Y, and Z?" To which I, or another, gets to say, "Well, these are some other options you might not have considered," and maybe this sparks hope.

Understanding this autonomy impacts success. And it might look different for everyone. We don't all have the same goals. Everyone has a different skillset. Maybe someone wants to be a manager, but that's not what he or she is best suited to. But here are ten thousand other things that you can do! Let's take a look at all of those.

It seems like such a simple thing to help people understand that there are options but we're up against deprogramming years of learned absolutes that are wrong. Learned helplessness is part of that. It's amazing. I still have people in my life, who can't decide on their own. Even if they've been around the (recovery meeting) rooms for twenty years or so. I understand the fear for users to go into their mind alone. It *is* a dangerous neighborhood. I've made plenty of mistakes, sober *and* while using.

For me, harm reduction has been about meeting myself where I was, and not leaving myself there. I've had to tell myself, "Keep stretching, keep growing." I've had to take a timeout, and kind of consolidate all the richness I had learned, and I've needed to use these experiences to make my way through to the next level. Having dreams is a part of life. Sadly, many of us have not been allowed to have that voice or to even have that dream.

I've learned the solution is to get more people to use their voice. Sometimes, this means pulling us as a society kicking and screaming into a new way of helping people connect with treatment. But that's where recovery resides: understanding that what's best for you might be what's right for them.

For me? *That* is what harm reduction is.

Njon can be reached at njon.sanders@gmail.com

EMANUEL SFERIOS

The first place I encountered harm reduction was at Berkeley Needle Exchange in the mid-1990s. I was an activist with Food Not Bombs, cooking and serving free meals in People's Park four days a week, and one of our collective members, John L., also worked with the local needle exchange program. He invited me to volunteer. I wasn't an IV drug user, but needle exchange made perfect sense to me. The drug war wasn't working, so why not help people use drugs more safely? I was 25 years old, and that's where I got my start.

I really became a full-time harm reductionist was when I founded DanceSafe in 1998. The story of how I started DanceSafe is interesting. To really explain it, I have to go back earlier, to when I first took ecstasy.

It was 1985 and I was a teenage runaway living in a warehouse in downtown St. Petersburg, Florida. I had met two adult Quakers who became mentors to me. They were activists, members of the American Friends Service Committee, and were really the first adults in my life who took an interest in me. One day, I was talking to them about my childhood trauma and one of them asked if I have ever considered therapy. Of course I hadn't. As a homeless teen, how could I afford it?

But then, coincidentally, a few weeks later I just happened to read the first ever article in a mainstream publication about MDMA, or ecstasy. The DEA had just announced they were going to ban it because people in Texas were using it in night-clubs. The article was mainly about a group of therapists who were suing the DEA to keep it legal, because, they said, it produced insights. "Five years of therapy in six hours," a therapist quoted in the article said. I thought, "Well, if I can't afford professional therapy, maybe I can do this drug."

It took me six months to find it. I remember asking all my friends, but none of them had even heard of ecstasy. This was 1985, keep in mind, before the rave culture got started. That fall I finally found someone who said he could get it for me. He drove me to a goth nightclub in Tampa called Masquerade. I gave him forty bucks and he told me to wait outside. Ten minutes later a woman comes out wearing all black. "Are you Manny?" she asks. I think she was more nervous selling drugs to a 15-year-old than I was buying them. After a short conversation she hands me two tablets and says, "Don't take more than one," and, "Here's my card if you want more."

The ecstasy tablets looked like chewable vitamin C pills—grey and wafer-shaped. I saved them for a few months and then one evening in early 1986 my best friend and I went to the beach and each took one. It was an amazing experience! I talked about things that had happened to me I never had told anyone before. I also remember, for the first time in my life, feeling love for myself. MDMA began a process of healing for me. I took it about a dozen times over the next few years and I can honestly say I would not be the person I am today without it.

So, now it's 1998 and I'm living in Berkeley. I had just gotten married and a friend of mine gives us two ecstasy tablets as a gift. I hadn't taken MDMA in a decade, and I wondered what we had learned about it in all this time. I got online and the first thing I came across was an article about how prohibition had created an adulterated market with counterfeit pills that were killing people. At the same time, the Dutch government— always three steps ahead of the rest of the world—had set up a program in Amsterdam where people could bring their ecstasy tablets in to get them spot tested using a chemical called Marquis reagent, which could weed out the counterfeit pills. I immediately decided I was going to do the same thing here. However, neither the Berkeley nor Haight-Ashbury free clinics would let me use their locations to set up testing centers, so I decided to go to raves to do the testing. Meet the people where they're at, literally. And that's how I became the first person in the world to provide drug checking in public spaces (we called it "ecstasy pill testing" back then.)

Other than to save lives, I started DanceSafe to honor MDMA, a drug that had been so important in my own personal healing. And another reason was because I realized that drug checking was a way to expand harm reduction to a much broader population. Back in 1998 harm reduction was pretty much just needle exchange, which came out of the HIV/AIDS movement. Which meant that it was widely perceived to only apply to gays and IV drug users. Now we suddenly had teenagers dying from counterfeit party drugs. I saw an opportunity to expand the concept of harm reduction to include drug checking. Test before you ingest. Little did I know that twenty-five years later, in the age of fentanyl, it would become a multi-million dollar industry!

I modeled DanceSafe on Food Not Bombs—a peer-based, grassroots activist organization I was working with at the time, that had chapters all over the world. Our chapter cooked and served food in People's Park five days a week. The motto of Food Not Bombs is, "Anyone can cook. Anyone can eat." In other words, we weren't a professional social service organization serving food to the so-called "homeless." Many of us were unhoused ourselves. We were simply people in the community helping each other, and we invited anyone to cook and eat with us. We were anarchists and activists and runaways, and we considered what we did "direct action." Several interesting people were involved, including those with various behavioral health issues. I saw how engaging in meaningful work—something as simple as cooking and serving food—could really empower people and improve their mental health, including my own. We all accepted and respected each other, no matter how different we all were.

So I founded DanceSafe on these same principles. We were drug users helping ourselves, helping our community. Under this model, there are no "others." Anyone who wanted to could get involved. We were people who used drugs and who believed we had a right to a safe supply. And if prohibition had created a dangerous, adulterated market, we were going to take matters into our own hands. We tested our pills and educated each other about safer drug use and safer partying.

To be honest, it was the rave community, the early volunteers, who made DanceSafe what it was. I was just a community organizer, new to the rave culture. I organized by empowering and encouraging others. Literally, for the entire first year there wasn't even a nonprofit entity. We were just people who cared—setting up booths with no official organization behind us. I didn't start the nonprofit until later when the work expanded to multiple cities. I realized that these autonomous groups needed protection. We were all using the same name (DanceSafe), and it dawned on me that if someone got arrested selling drugs behind the booth, for example, or did something else criminal or unethical, it could hurt everyone. So I incorporated the national nonprofit and then required each group or chapter to sign a name-licensing agreement. You can use the name DanceSafe as long as you agree to a minimum set of responsibilities. These included proper pill testing procedures. Never tell someone their ecstasy tablet was "good, pure or safe." No drug use is 100% safe. Just give them the results of the test. It's always up to them whether to consume the pill or not. It was a basic liability contract simply to protect all the chapters. Other than these minimal requirements to use the name, the chapters remained independent and autonomous. This grassroots model lasted more than twenty years, until a few years ago when the current board and national office staff centralized the organization. Today DanceSafe chapters are no longer autonomous. The national nonprofit flies people to festivals from around the country, and tries to get them to read scripts. It isn't peer-based drug education anymore, which makes me sad. But I can proudly say that during the two decades when we were a real, bottom-up, grassroots movement, we changed the party drug culture in the US. It's a testament to people power, and proof that people who use drugs care about their health and safety.

What is harm reduction? I think many of us would probably say it includes any positive step forward. That's certainly one of the definitions, but there's plenty of others too. To me, harm reduction encompasses risk reduction. It's ultimately about being responsible when you use drugs. Every drug has a different safety profile and risk-to-benefit profile. Not to mention drugs affect people differently. There's no cookie-cutter, one-size-fits-all approach to any drug. Some people can take higher doses of a particular drug, and use it more often without developing problematic use. There are a ton of factors involved. A big part of harm reduction to me is non-judgmentalism. In the music culture, that often necessitates conversations about what I call psychedelic chauvinism, the idea that psychedelics are "good drugs" and don't deserve the stigma put on other drugs (the "bad drugs"). But There are no good or bad drugs. There are just drugs. And the answer to stigma is to get rid of it completely, for all drugs, not to try to elevate some (the ones you personally like) above others. In other words, let's not throw opioid users under the bus! Remember, the vast majority of people who use *any* drug don't do so problematically. This includes meth and opioids. People need to know this so they don't judge others. I think this is really important.

Anti-drug culture manifests the very abusive drug taking behavior it claims to be preventing. The best thing we can do to save lives is to end the judgment and stigma. That means we need to respect people who use drugs. We need to go beyond compassion, and include respect, because compassion can still embody an element of judgmentalism. "Oh, those poor people," that kind of thing. Drug users need respect more than they need compassion. People treated with respect are more capable of making better decisions for themselves.

For a long time I had a vision of a future for harm reduction that centered around legal regulation. I still think we should keep that in mind and talk about it. If drugs are legally regulated, there would be no need for drug checking because quality control would be built into the system, like it is with alcohol. It would look different than the way we regulate alcohol, but it's really what we need. For example, we need heroin maintenance. Not just methadone and bupe (buprenorphine). Or how about opioid-of-choice maintenance? Help people who choose to use opioids do so safely. I really think this is the only way we're going to save lives given how ubiquitous fentanyl is today. Unregulated fentanyl is simply too dangerous. Yet, it's the only opioid in town, and so we have more than a hundred thousand people a year dying now. And it's only going to get worse. If people had a safe supply of safer opioids, and if we helped them manage their use with doctors and nurses in clinics, we could shrink the fentanyl market. Probably not eliminate it, but dramatically shrink it. Is this realistic? Is our country ready for a safe supply of regulated opioids? We can't even get single payer healthcare in this country. How are we going to get government funding for such highly stigmatized medicine?

I'll keep shouting from my soap box, but I guess after thirty years in the movement, I've come to the conclusion that the most I'll see in my lifetime is decriminalization. If we can get decriminalization, that will result in two really important things. One, the public conversation will open up. People will no longer be afraid to talk openly about their drug use. They will be able to talk to teachers, doctors, and even police, without fear of arrest. And second, it will open up public space for harm reduction services, like drug checking, which are already starting to become more popular. For the first seventeen years DanceSafe used to be the only drug checking program around. Now we have programs starting up in many cities, which serves as a type of quality control. It's a band-aid measure, especially when it comes to fentanyl, but it's a start. And decriminalization will also usher in other types of harm reduction services.

Harm reduction has come a long way for sure, but the professionalization of harm reduction has been a double-edged sword. Maybe as little as ten years ago—definitely twenty-five years ago when I started DanceSafe—all of us harm reductionists were activists. We did it because we knew people who died, and we didn't want to die ourselves. Now, a lot of people doing the work are professionals, hired by state and country programs, or by large nonprofits with grant money. This even includes DanceSafe. And many of the people working the jobs today were never activists. They may mean well, but when a movement turns into a profession, fewer people are willing to rock the boat. There's less "pushing the envelope," so to speak, when it entails risking your career. So we have fewer harm reductionists today advocating for heroin maintenance than we did 20 years ago. There's a lot of money in harm reduction now. Millions of dollars for naloxone and fentanyl test strips and jobs. And that's a good thing. But the cost comes in the professionalization, which tends to preserve the status quo.

We need a big push. We need a push for heroin maintenance and for other, new solutions. This becomes more difficult when a movement becomes professionalized. I'll give you an example. My friends jokingly call me the king of fentanyl test strips, because I was the first person to perform laboratory studies assessing their use for harm reduction, and I'm basically the person who popularized their use. And now there's a giant industry surrounding them. Federal and state grant money pays for tens of millions of strips a year. They're being distributed everywhere. But fentanyl test strips are not the solution to the opioid crisis. For one, they're only helpful for non-opioid users, who want to make sure there's no fentanyl contaminating their stimulants or party drugs. They're no longer helpful for opioid users for the simple reason that fentanyl is *everywhere*. For many years now in the US, it has almost entirely replaced heroin. If you're an opioid user, you know you're using fentanyl. There's no need to test for fentanyl. Fentanyl is the only game in town. What might help is a test for how strong your fentanyl is. A quantitative test. People are dying because unregulated fentanyl can be anywhere from 3% to 30% pure or even higher—people have no idea how strong their pills or powders are before consuming them. I'm working with a German company right now to develop a quantitative fentanyl test, or "QTest" as we call them. We have them for a few other drugs, and they can give the user the percent purity or strength of their pills or powders before they consume them. I think such a test would save far more lives than fentanyl test strips, because most of the people dying today are people intentionally using fentanyl; they simply take too much because they don't know how strong their baggie is. Are we ready as a culture to help people use fentanyl more safely? Fentanyl test strips have become widely accepted (and funded) I believe precisely because they help people who want to avoid using fentanyl. That's become accepted because we demonize fentanyl. It's bad and so sure, let's help people avoid it. But people who think that way should not kid themselves that fentanyl test strips are even taking a dent out of the opioid crisis. They're not. A fentanyl QTest might, and in the process actually save a lot of lives. We would need to accept that we are helping people use fentanyl more safely. Are we ready to do that? (I am.)

I really want people to understand that the vast majority of people who use drugs are making an intentional choice that benefits them, and that harm reduction should respect that choice. If, as a culture, we keep pretending that drugs are only (or even primarily) harmful, and that all we can do is help these poor people reduce the harm they are inevitably doing to themselves by using drugs, then we're never going to make progress saving lives and improving public health. To me, everything comes back to stigma and judgment. We need to respect people who use drugs and then help them use those drugs as safely as possible.

Emanuel can be reached at GrassrootsHarmReduction.org

CHRIS STEIL

After our work together (*Kicking and Screaming*, first ed.), and later taking alcohol and other drug classes (AOD), things changed for me. I saw that the model of drug treatment was moving towards harm reduction rather than 12 Step. I also had no idea that in the future I would be dealing with sponsees or mentees that were in reduction programs, that I would be challenged with working with them. They needed help, and I'm in the business of help, so I had to change *my* way. I was challenged in trying to figure out how 12 Step and complete abstinence fit in with harm reduction, coming to where this person is—where the guy I'm working with is. I have to adapt in whatever ways I can: lifestyle, mental emotional condition, recovery condition, looking at that sponsee in these areas and not just asking "are they using?" In other words, where is this person in their recovery? Are they in recovery (by their definition)? Are they new? Or are they totally strung out? Do they need drugs to have sex? Does recovery mean you don't get to have sex anymore because you don't use drugs? Is he using drugs and having dangerous sex? I could keep going. Harm reduction required I look at his life in many ways and ask totally different questions [than I had been].

Talking about harm reduction in counseling sessions and DAC classes, I was being exposed to harm reduction quite a bit. I began to realize that even as I stayed in and participated in my own 12 Step recovery process, there needed to be other workable models [to use for recovery]. I also noticed how people I knew and respected either weren't finding 12 Step workable or applicable to their lives. And sometimes they were finding abusive people hiding in the Fellowships.

In my AA meetings, I found that some people accepted abuse as a rite of passage. They were saying things to newcomers like, "You have to take the cotton out of your ears and put it in your mouth," or "Maybe you're not done [using drugs] yet." I was also hearing lots of, "You can't take those [medications]. We don't take anything in this program. Nothing!" And some of us needed something (like prescription antidepressants) to stave off the symptoms of clinical depression because we were just hurting too much. And 12 Step couldn't handle that. The people there said, "This program is about complete abstinence, period." 12 Step folks just couldn't handle the idea that someone might have to take the edge off of either mental or emotional or pain issues, or just the fact that life can be such a shithole sometimes. And finally, we couldn't handle hearing, "Maybe I need drugs to have good sex." Yeah, me and 12 Step didn't know how to deal with that either!

To me, harm reduction is *with intent*, to use the least amount of the least harmful substance(s) to make life acceptable. No pressure. I also think it's about making oneself available and open to getting help and healthier ideas. I see a counselor, a doctor, and I eat healthy. That's all harm reduction. Harm reduction is also clean needles, safer sex, improvements in your living situation. And all of this takes into account that the person we're working with has to be able to do those things. The challenge is that when I'm using, I get wasted, I'm psychotic and I'm in "animal mode," so all that stuff that might make using "safer" is off the table. When I'm living like an animal, I'm thinking like an animal. All I want is more dope and basically what I want is the "yet." That's *my* addiction. I want the end result (feeling from the drug).

For me, another part of practicing harm reduction is trying to listen and participate with people attempting to improve themselves. I also think of my harm reduction as keeping myself safe from emotional and physical distress. Thinking about all that pretty much made me remember I had my jaw broken a while back by a sponsee. (I need to be careful when I try to meet people where they are, to make sure they can't get in a right hook!) I don't want to become part of their problem or part of their delusions. I'm there to help but not if you don't want it, at least not right now.

To me the other part of harm reduction is on the commercial, industrial, and societal level, which I don't think I can discuss well. I feel a bit hopeless about our society and the human race, okay? And what *that* means is that when we talk about needle [exchange] places and more, it's a societal problem. That's the big problem. It's mental and emotional problems due to outside societal forces—not just because of substance abuse. And our society would rather brush us off the fucking table. *We* must direct resources—delegate resources—major resources toward these problems. I think halfway houses are probably way cheaper than going out and trying to provide care for the homeless, right? What I mean is right now we have homeless from all over the place in all different kinds of condition and needs. And we need to look at more than just homelessness. All of this is to say that what I think harm reduction needs is more literature and resources on what's working and what isn't working. We need to continue to support and accept safer using sites as well as places to bathe and get a change of clothes. And there's still the issue of someone going animalistic or becoming really anti-social. These things can happen when someone's homelessness, addiction and degradation are at such a deep level. Homelessness, harm reduction, addiction need to be our big picture.

I wish people knew that harm reduction isn't a license to use freely, without intention. That's what a lot of people in my 12 Step arenas think, even some that were in the business of using and who are now counselors—but that's not the case. Harm reduction, like any recovery model, requires work and intention. Once again, it's the same people who think that it's just a free license to use, a free-for-all. You know, you have to do *something*. Even my friends who have left 12 Step are still doing *something*—something spiritual, something social, something charitable, something to keep the heart going and [and body] to stay clean. Finally, lots of people don't realize that harm reduction expands into the industry—in other words, the Recovery Industry. Society-wide scale is needed—changes in practices and attitudes. Change is needed on the sidewalk and in city hall, okay?

But in the bigger picture, what do we do as a society to expand harm reduction? And what and how do we spread the word of what harm reduction means? As a society, I think we still think of harm reduction on the individual level—reduction of harm to the individual—but it's also harm reduction to society. Yeah, the less harm done to society, the less spent on medical, psychiatric, and judicial maladies, then resources can be spent in other ways to improve society. Well, that is, if we're really intent on helping each other. And that's all I got.

Chris can be reached at c3steil@gmail.com

MAIA SZALAVITZ

Thankfully, harm reduction found me. I was injecting drugs in New York City during the eighties at a time when half the people injecting drugs were already HIV positive. One day, I was hanging out at a friend's house. He'd left to cop, so it was just me and another woman who was there trying to get him into rehab. This was going to be his little last hurrah. And you have to have one, right? So, I was just talking to this woman, whom I'd never met. I was about to shoot up and she said to me, "Y'know, if you're going to shoot up with used needles, you need to clean them with bleach." I considered myself a pretty informed person. I watched the TV news, read the paper. But I had no idea that HIV affected IV drug users. The big story was the disease's impact on gay men. I thought, "Well, I'm not a gay man. I don't need to worry." But I was wrong.

I learned to protect myself very rapidly after that. I always used bleach or didn't share. And so thankfully I did not get infected. But I was furious that nobody was giving us this information. The impact of HIV on intravenous users wasn't the prominent narrative. It was as if people actually wanted to suppress it.

"Let the junkies die and send a message to the "good kids." The whole idea that one life was more valuable, or that another was more expendable, seemed horrible to me.

This is what led me to reaching out and meeting people heading the harm reduction movement at the time. I also got into 12 Step recovery, about two years after I was taught to use clean needles. In 12 Step, there was such an opposition to harm reduction, which fed off this whole "enabling" business. I never bought into that idea (i.e., that harm reduction is enabling people to keep using drugs) but I did buy into a lot of stuff because I was told the 12 Steps was the only path to recovery, and I was desperate to recover. By the time I got to rehab, I had people telling me there's a 90% chance of relapse. I didn't understand how treatment providers could be telling us that 90% would slip and yet not be committed to protecting those people? And the way to protect those people would involve harm reduction.

I grew infuriated that treatment centers and proponents of abstinence opposed syringe exchange, these measures designed to ease suffering and help drug users stay alive. From my first introduction to harm reduction, I was in favor of it for this reason.

When I finally got into recovery, I figured, "Okay, well, I've always wanted to be a writer. I can do that! Let's see how much information I can help get out there." That basically became my career. My writing career coincided with the start of the harm reduction movement too. I got to talk to most of the earliest pioneers of it. At least on the East Coast.

There were conferences. The internet was beginning. One of the ways I became a true harm reductionist was via an internet list, where all of that abstinence-only stuff got pounded out of me. I never opposed needle exchange, but I'd been taught that abstinence was the only path to a better life. All of these mistaken ideas I had about the nature of addiction I was forced to confront, challenge. I don't like being wrong, so I changed.

There's a terrific quote by a famous economist, maybe it's Keynes or one of Galbraith's, something like "When the facts change, I change my mind. What do you do?" The facts changed. I changed my mind. I wanted to understand addiction. I wanted to understand why we would let people die needless deaths from HIV. Why do we just see people with addiction as such bad people? None of it made sense.

I discovered I had learned a ton of myths about addiction, both from school and from being on the street, and then from rehab. It wasn't until I started really looking at the scientific literature that I began to appreciate a multidisciplinary approach. If you only factor in the biology or examine the psychology or only look at the sociology, you are missing big pieces. Also, understanding history is paramount, because racism has dictated some *horrible* policies. It's sad but true. Race *does* factor into so much of how we treat addiction. Many of our policies don't reduce addiction nor even reduce drug use. Often, they produce the opposite effect: hopelessness, gangs, etc. If your goal is actually locking up Black and Brown people? Sure, the drug war is pretty effective! Once you accept that our policy is not about drugs, but rather getting people elected by using racist tropes, you begin to see why we are not treating addiction in terms of its real-world implications and ramifications. People come into the drug policy area, and think, "Wow. This is a stupid, illogical mess." And they're not wrong! The answers are pretty simple about what *would* work. Why aren't we doing them? Then you run into the whole racism and politics thing, and you're like, "Oh, yeah, that's why."

Some things *have* changed. Several aspects proved to be critical for that to happen. One of the most important was Michelle Alexander's book, *The New Jim Crow*. Sadly, many Black community leaders initially supported prohibition and the whole crack down/lock them up approach. They didn't really see any alternative to the devasting effects of drug use in their communities. Drug policy reformers in the 1980's seemed like out of touch white people who wanted to get stoned and didn't care about Black communities. There was a disconnect. Dr. Alexander's book challenged these beliefs, and she did an enormous amount of intellectual work speaking around the country to spread the word.

With the rise of the internet, people could actually get accurate information about drugs which, through the mainstream media, wasn't always an option. Sure, you could go to a library and do your own research. But the internet provided that same information with the click of a mouse (which beats two bus transfers and a half mile walk to your local library). I mean, how many people are going to make the effort to learn this stuff when they think they already know about it from the media?

Online, the legalization and harm reduction side had the prohibitionist side beat by the number of people represented. The early adopters of the internet were deadheads, libertarians, nerds, academics. Before the prohibitionists caught on, there were more of *us* than there were of *them*. And now, more people have started seeing through a lot of nonsense—like the racial inequality of sentencing, how there can't be only *one* path to recovery—but we have lots of disinformation and misinformation out there. Which is also due to the same invention that's helped educate: the internet.

Back in the day, I had a letter published in the *New England Journal of Medicine*, because they ran this article that said, basically, "Oh, my God, people are getting drug information on the internet from these biased sites, and they should be going to the objective government sites!" And I was, like, seriously? The objective government site? The one that touts racist policies and is clueless about how to treat addiction? I mean, PubMed is fine but I can't encourage getting your drug info from the DEA website!

Another example: There is solid research showing a 50% reduction in all-cause mortality if patients can stay on methadone or buprenorphine. Preventing that information from being available to the masses is, literally, deadly. There are still going to be plenty of people who will refuse such medications for whatever reason. (Often users will get into recovery and be adamant about not being on *any* drug.) And that should be an absolute individual choice. However, it should be made in the context of having that information about how such medications help, and not because they've been brow-beaten that abstinence is superior. It comes down to what first helps keep someone alive.

One of the things that I think people really don't understand about the use of methadone and buprenorphine is they can be used for abstinence—or for sheer harm reduction. The main point is that some people are going to continue to use while taking methadone or buprenorphine. But they also benefit from being in touch with services and getting access to counseling. They benefit from maintaining tolerance, so they are less likely to die of overdose. And if it means that for one day they don't have to play Russian roulette and score fentanyl, that's a win. If they don't have to experience physical withdrawal that day, that's a win.

Of course, ideally, you want people to attend high quality counseling. That will help them make healthy changes. But making *everybody* get those services just to get the medication is ridiculous. It also doesn't help people who just don't need counseling anymore. These barriers undermine harm reduction.

I define harm reduction as any policy that focuses, first, on stopping people from getting hurt, rather than stopping them from getting high. And then all the humanistic, lovely stuff comes in once you make protecting people's lives and health the priority, because you have to treat them with dignity, you have to recognize that their lives count. You have to, you know, include all the stuff about meeting people where they are because I think that some of the definitions, they sound great, and they do represent what's going on in harm reduction, but they don't explain to people what the *point* is, or how you got from here to there. But when you just say we're focusing on stopping harms, not stopping highs, then I think it's automatically less controlling. What we're caring about is what society and government *should* care about: are people getting hurt or not? I don't think government should be in my business about whether I'm getting euphoria. I do recognize that if I am hurting myself or others, then society has an interest in that. But I don't think there's an interest in the whole, "Oh, my God, you might get pleasure. What if you're naturally born with extra endorphins or something? You're not gonna—you can't—police that!" You can try, but it really doesn't work.

I think the future has to be understanding that harm reduction is not just needle exchange. It's not just naloxone. It's not just working with people who are actively using; it is a policy thing. For example, some people *need* opiates for a condition. If someone is being over-prescribed opioids that are harming them, you want to fix that, but the idea that you'll just cut everybody off is as stupid as it is harmful.

The broader policy must encompass harm reduction. And for ourselves and the work we do, we must also consider personal temperament. Are you somebody who wants to work within the system? Are you comfortable there? Or are you somebody who'd prefer a more radical approach? Because we need both: people trying to change the system from within and people outside helping those in the system to envision extreme change.

When we listen to *all* those voices, we have a better chance of representing everyone who needs to be represented. We want to be inclusive, not exclusive. We also can't be arguing over what represents progress—"I'm more PC than you are," or "I'm more woke than you are"—that stuff really needs to go. We need *everyone*—even people we disagree with on some issues.

The term "harm reduction" has also been misrepresented to mean nothing but overdose prevention sites, safe injection facilities. People get scared of harm reduction, including syringe exchange, because they think that's *all* there is to it, that nothing else is being done to improve the lives of people who use drugs. And that couldn't be more wrong. The idea of meeting people, treating them humanly—accepting them for where they are and not where *you* want them to be—it empowers people, which in turn allows them to be more capable of change. When you treat somebody kindly and respectfully as a full human, they begin to believe they are worthwhile, worthy of a better life, and they will often learn to take those first steps themselves if they see the destination as being achievable and worth the journey.

And that is where you can actually see change, the kind of change even the abstinence-only people want, because people who use drugs start to see a different path is possible. If they know what they are doing or how they are living isn't working, or they say to themselves, "I have tried controlling this, it's not working. I need to do something different." At that point, if they are engaged in a harm reduction program, we have a real shot at making a difference. We absolutely need to thread harm reduction throughout our treatment system. And to do that, we *must* get rid of all of the confrontational and humiliating aspects in the industry, where patients are made to feel as though they are "bad" or "weak" people.

People don't believe me that when I tell them what treatment is often really like. I'll hear, "You just oppose treatment because you're into harm reduction." I say to them, "No, I want treatment to be respectful." We're talking about a highly traumatized population of people. If you're going to put them into a situation that is guaranteed to re-traumatize them, then, no, I can't support that. But respectful, humane care? I absolutely support treatment that looks like that.

It's sad, but if you want to make your success rates look good as a treatment provider, you can just be really mean to people. Get the people who aren't fully committed to recovery or have really complex trauma or mental illness to drop out. Then you can say, "Look! Our graduates have an 80% success rate!" But have you actually helped 80% of the people that walked in the door? Hell no. Because most of them walked right out.

Right now, it's imperative for people to understand that our treatment system is in peril and needs a major overhaul. That doesn't mean I am against programs that want you to be abstinent. I think we need all types of care, for all types of people, and we need choices. But we can't make perfection the enemy of progress.

Maia can be reached at http://maiasz.com

LORIE VIOLETTE

My introduction to harm reduction began when I started volunteering for a syringe service program. At the time, I was attending our local junior college. Given my interests in helping others, my counselor suggested I look into outreach programs. But I didn't know anything about outreach! My counselor saw what I couldn't—namely, that my personality was perfectly suited for it. I applied for a couple positions. One of them was for HIV prevention, and involved working with people who used drugs. I thought, "Oh, my goodness, I don't know about this"—I don't have a history of substance use, nothing serious anyway. I'd tried some drugs, but haven't had any issues in my life. I was interested in learning about it, because my parents were both substance users. My dad used heroin. I remember watching him inject heroin. I was a young kid. And then my parents separated, and I learned my mom also used, but she was into uppers, and so she did a lot of methamphetamine. When you look at it like that, I guess it makes sense they wouldn't stay together. Talk about opposite ends of the spectrum! I saw both sides, up close and personal. Even though I didn't make the connection, the counselor who suggested I work in that field clearly did.

Still, I didn't understand much about addiction, and even less about harm reduction, which in those days was really in its infancy. Initially, the needle exchange program where I volunteered was in an alley, behind a local community market. I would show up every Friday at 4 p.m., bagging supplies and getting prepared. I'd make little cartoons, advertising about all the services we offered. I loved it—I loved helping people without preaching or trying to dictate what their life should be. I was there as an equal. I wasn't there to tell these people they were "bad" or even try to persuade them to change. I met them where they were at, at that moment, providing a service they needed, and helping keep them safe.

This part-time position soon turned into a full-time job. It was so rewarding. It felt good treating people with dignity and respect, these men and women as they were, and not as I wanted them to be. That wasn't my call to make. The choice to use or not use belongs to the individual. I was there to help them stay alive. If they chose to keep using, I wanted to assist their doing so safely. And if someone expressed interest in getting help, I was there for that too. I'd direct folks toward other services, whatever that may be. Inpatient, outpatient, meetings. I was trained to help with that, which for me was very fulfilling.

Coming at this from my parents' substance use, I only understood chaos. I didn't know what was going on in our house. Part of that was, yes, I was young, but when I began working in the field, working one-on-one with patients, I realized that my parents were also dealing with many of these struggles. Understanding and accepting that helped me heal and move on. Outreach work filled my heart. I'd say to myself, "I'm doing the right thing." I could see I was providing a valuable service. Of course, I've also had people say, "Why would I help these people?" Meaning, why would I enable self-destructive behavior? As a harm reductionist, we take these insults with a grain of salt, and just keep moving and doing what we do. We've heard it all.

Growing up with parents who used, I experienced a world many don't. When I became a teenager, I got involved with boyfriends who were drug dealers. Some boyfriends were abusive. Some were pimps. I wasn't aware what that meant! I was living with this street mentality, but I was still growing up, young and inexperienced. I got turned out at a very young age—meaning boyfriends would persuade me into having sex with men for money. I thought that my making money for them was helping our relationship. I didn't have anyone looking out for my best interests. Now I see the harm reduction in the sex work arena. It all intersects—sex, drugs, runaways, mental health, domestic violence—everything in the world crosses paths, impacting another.

People often ask me how I feel about my parents, and their using and introducing me to that world. Honestly, I have a great deal of compassion. To this day, my dad still suffers from substance use disorder. He's also managed to sustain prolonged periods of sobriety. But he's human. Life throws us curveballs. For the last ten years, my father has been actively using, and I have a relationship with him. We have a good relationship. Of course, it's difficult to watch someone you love suffer. My father suffers in lots of ways. I've helped him with supplies, making sure he has sterile works. That's what we do as harm reductionists, right? I feel blessed that he's comfortable enough to ask me. Because I'd rather that, than having him using non-sterile works, getting sick, and dying.

My mom passed away early this year. She had been not using hard drugs for twenty, thirty years. Yeah, she smoked pot on a regular basis, but I don't look at that as a substance use disorder. Especially compared to how she used to be. I have one half-sister (same dad), who struggled with many of the same issues as our father, but she got through it. We all have to take our own road, and we finish the race in our own time. The key to harm reduction is keeping folks alive until they are ready to move onto the next phase of their lives. I later worked for another needle exchange-type organization, which also involved HIV testing and outreach. This was a bigger organization, with an abstinence-based treatment philosophy and program. But they had a health services component added to their larger program (the department that I worked in), which did have a methadone clinic. There was also a youth program and they had a residential program. A little bit of everything. This is really where I got my feet wet, especially in regards to HIV awareness and AIDS prevention.

Fast forward to where I began working with Megan Murphy at Face to Face. She and I worked very closely together to kick-start an HIV-testing component. And I helped them get that going. I helped provide trainings and was there on site, once a week, to conduct the testing. And so we kind of began this relationship. The first time I met her—this would've been in 2009—Megan said to me, "This is where you're destined to work." She was right! In 2016, I started my journey at Face to Face. We were out in the open, publicly recognized. When Face to Face began, they were operating underground. Since I've arrived, Face to Face has actually become certified as a syringe service program! We got our seal of approval from the great state of California! And we've been providing services, loud, proud, and out in the open since. We are currently the largest syringe service program in Sonoma County. Wow! We exchanged something like, 850,000 syringes last year. Crazy! We are the syringe exchange program that folks come to for help. There are other programs in our county, but their hours are very limited. We're open—*very* open! We actually have a mobile unit, a van that drives around, looking for folks who need our help, seeking out those in need. Kinda like the Batmobile! One of the silver linings of the pandemic: it highlighted our need to be mobile. We can't always wait for the afflicted to come to us. Sometimes we're going to need to go to them. Face to Face saw that need. So we went out to find a van and secure some funding for this. And now we have a van. It's called "On the Move."

Harm reduction comes in many shapes and sizes, some stationary, some very much on the go. I'll often hear volunteers expressing shock. They'll say stuff like, "Oh my goodness! I didn't realize that this encompasses so much." It does. I didn't get that at first either, but I've been in harm reduction most of my life. If I had to whittle harm reduction's governing principle, I'd say it comes down to accepting people—accepting them for who they are. That's the only way for us to see what they need; it's the only way to help them succeed. It's difficult to provide these services if you're preoccupied judging lifestyles or choices. Being judgmental is antithetical to compassion; it's saying I know more than you about your life, so you should listen to me. Which is very hard for another adult to hear and act on. They will react as though they are being attacked, which in turn will cause them to get defensive, and then where are you? They are still out there, using. Your judgment has only made their lives and lots harder.

This brings us back to the concept of "enabling." There's a very vocal school out there in the recovery community that says un-less you're convincing addicts to completely abstain, you are pro-longing their sickness. But many substance users aren't there yet. Our mission is to keep them safe so that when (if) the time should come, they'll have a fighting chance. When a person begins us-ing drugs, they might not know how to inject themselves properly. You think that's going to stop them? No! They'll do it anyway, and by not, say, using an alcohol wipe to sterilize the injection site, they are running the risk of infections and worse. That is a taboo topic. Do we want to show an addict how to inject themselves properly? Like I say, a user is going to use if he or she wants to, and by setting up these barriers, drawing this hard line in the sand that claims only prohibition works, you're erecting harmful barri-ers. People won't feel safe asking for help in such an environment. You want a user to see you and say, "Okay, I'm in a safe place to talk." And I trust what this person is going to share with me. We don't want walls built up. We want walls torn down.

Being consistent with your messaging, consistent with what you're doing—it breaks barriers, brings down these walls, and helps empower people to make those changes—regardless of what that change may be. It could be anything—changing healthcare providers, visiting the dentist, making an offer on a house. Life requires self-esteem to survive. How could we ex-pect someone who's been told how awful they are and wrong they've been to just turn it around? It's like we expect them to give up these drugs they've been relying on to make it through the day, and suddenly they'll be whole, happy, fulfilled, and full of self-confidence? The human mind doesn't work like that. So much of recovery involves a person's self-esteem and how they feel. And if they feel horrible about themselves, they will never find a place where they feel comfortable, like they belong, or are wanted. At the end of the day, people need to feel loved and accepted for who they are.

There's not a stereotypical syringe exchange participant. It's not like you see in the movies. Not every user is pushing a cart or diving in a dumpster. Sure, some fit those stereotypes. But drug use covers a much broader swath. It's our grandmas. It's our grandpas, our kids. It's our school teachers. Nobody is immune to it. And it's eye opening to see some of the folks that walk through the door to receive supplies and services and we offer. One size fits all doesn't apply to recovery or users.

Our number one goal is safety. We offer two types of Narcan, the intramuscular variety, and the nasal kind. Each requires different administration, including how much to use. We provide Narcan. We also teach how to use it. We also provide fentanyl test strips. For me, fentanyl test strips and Narcan go together. We've realized we need to start educating folks about what an overdose looks like. The main piece may involve Narcan to keep them breathing. A person who has overdosed also needs to be conscious, alert, and awake.

Face to Face is a "big-picture" organization, covering all facets of those living with addiction. We offer non-medical case management to people living with HIV. And Face to Face helps house people. There's financial assistance for vital necessities, like heat and food. We help getting public aid with utilities like PG& E. For many, just having basic needs met presents a challenge. It's, like, "Whoa, I just woke up this morning, and I didn't get to brush my teeth or have breakfast, but I gotta go to my appointment over here, right?" That's human nature. We want to ease burdens, not magnify them. I think building a rapport with that person, providing consistency you're there for them—

that's the key.

To me, this is harm reduction. My definition of the term: showing love and compassion, laced with hope, laced with caring, laced with support. Regardless. That's how I look at it, and that's how I present it. One day I'd like to see safe injection sites. Hopefully, funding and support of that will come through. In the meantime, my job is to be an advocate for and to help people—should they choose to use. I'm out there to help drug users be as safe and cared for as possible.

Lorie can be reached at lviolette@f2f.org

PART 2

"BOOTS ON THE GROUND"
OUTREACH WORKERS

MIKE BROWN

I was an IV opiate and meth user for many years. I started improving my health and wellness (which is my preferred definition of recovery) in 2017. My pathway included cannabis and suboxone. That's when I found my way into recovery advocacy. I just love helping people, and wanted to turn all that pain into purpose. I began with helping people connect with treatment resources around the country. Within a year though, I realized how dirty, dangerous, and shady the treatment industry can be. I couldn't do it, and had to leave. Aside from the shady things that were going on daily and how dangerous it is—traditional abstinence-only treatment options go completely against what I believe in.

I got in touch with Jamie Favaro, who heads NEXT Distro in NY. She sent me a few hundred Naloxone kits to start distributing, and I quickly found that harm reduction was my purpose.

In August of 2019, I started the world's first official, virtual overdose prevention service, called Never Use Alone. When I first started it, I honestly didn't think it would work. I didn't think anyone would trust us enough to call. Then in February 2020, the COVID lockdowns started, and the phone started ringing. As of August 2024, we've now taken fifty thousand calls, and we've alerted EMS to a callers location in 180 occasions! It's definitely working!

It's crazy how many in the recovery community have attacked me for it though. It's always the 12 Steppers—"You're enabling them," "You're encouraging drug use." It's amazing how fast people forget where they came from and what it was like. If they quit yesterday, they think everyone else should have quit yesterday, too.

It's like, "Come back when you're ready." People *are* ready. They just might not be ready for *your* philosophies or approach. If you make someone feel unwelcome, why would they want to come back and ask for your help? Then you have the NA doctors pushing people to get off of their medications so that they can have "real recovery" (whatever the hell that is). When they follow that dangerous advice and die, the NA doctor always says the same thing. "He (or she) just wasn't ready." No, you killed them! I often wonder if they feel guilt, or if the program has fooled them into believing that they really aren't at fault?

There was a guy in my home group. He had like twenty-five years or something of sobriety at the time. They were all about their recovery time, wearing it like rank on a uniform. This guy was basically the general in the meeting. The General decided that anybody on any psych meds or any medication of any kind—even over the counter, cold medicine or whatever—made one's recovery invalid. I know of *three* people he pushed to get off of their psych medications—to stop their Suboxone—and shortly thereafter two of these people died of overdose, and another committed suicide. And he's still there, this guy, this anointed General, with his twenty-five years. Still sitting in the rooms being praised. Like a hero. That's when I decided that I couldn't be a part of any program that is openly shaming, harming, and even killing the people they're supposed to be helping.

I found a pamphlet from the 2016 NA World Services that called people who were on MAT (Medication-Assisted Treatment) "active addicts." Despite MAT-based programs having far better success rates than most programs—including NA and AA. Yet, there are so many NA members that don't even know what their program's position is on MAT. They always say, "It's an outside issue" (an AA term), or "if it's prescribed, it's okay." That's not what NA actually believes though. They say that prescribed medications are okay—unless it's a medication that treats SUD. Then, they refer to them as "still using addicts" and they don't allow them to speak in a meeting.

It's the contradictory nonsense that gets me. 12 Steppers will be preaching at you about abstinence from all mood and mind-altering substances while they're drinking their fifth cup of coffee and smoking their tenth cigarette since the meeting ended.

That was part of the appeal of harm reduction. It's transparency, and embracing of the reality of the situation. For some, abstinence just isn't possible. It's nice to see a set of principles and values that are evidence-based. Care and compassion without compromise. Love and acceptance. Understanding and connection. The term represents different things to different people. But for me, personally, that's what harm reduction boils down to: an evidence-based approach to help reduce the risks associated with certain behaviors. It can be applied to somebody with an eating disorder, or substance use disorder.

A gambling problem, or anger issues. Seatbelts, helmets, parachutes—those are harm reduction! Sure, parachutes is an extreme example, and fewer people take exception to, say, advocating helmets for kids. People seem to only be against those harm reduction measures when they are focused on drug use. I think a lot of that comes from the DARE program. We're teaching kids from a very young age that drug users are bad people. These kids grow up, become parents, and it's still so ingrained. Conversely, I think the program often had the opposite effect on some kids: it made drugs seem alluring. A lot of studies have shown that. Yet, proponents of DARE and programs like it are still hanging on to that idea that it's going to help.

It doesn't make any sense how that we *still* have the War on Drugs, which authorities maintain is designed to keep people from destroying their lives with drug use—yet the penalties for being a drug-user often cause far more destruction of people's lives. The war on people who use drugs destroys your life so the drugs don't have to, basically. But, it brings in tons of money for the legal system! From their point of view, it's working perfectly. It's got nothing to do with keeping people safe, and everything to do with racism and corruption.

It's just nonsense, what's we've been tricked into believing. For example, how and why has the US managed to separate alcohol and drugs as if they are two separate things? We instinctively say "drugs *and* alcohol" as if they're two separate things! Cigarettes and alcohol are legal—and among the most dangerous drugs out there. Yet, they're socially acceptable. Why? Because they're legal. We don't bat an eye at they're use. We even promote the use of alcohol.

Here in Tennessee, cannabis isn't legal. But that's what helped me—cannabis. That was my form of MAT. Cannabis is what helped me stop shooting heroin and meth. But I spent all those years in the rooms thinking that cannabis use was failure. I would get a couple of months under my belt, I'd smoke a joint, and my sponsor would tell me how I screwed up, and had start all over. Well, Shhiitt! If I had to start over *anyway*, I might as well do what I *really* liked, and I'd end up with a needle in my arm, nearly dying of an overdose. All over a joint!?

AA and NA have such a stranglehold on the recovery industry, and they've earned this reputation that they really don't deserve. In the hundred years of the program, AA and NA enjoy a reputation of perfection. People—including our esteemed courts—believe that it works 100% of the time. And if it doesn't? Well, that's because you didn't work the program correctly. That you're "constitutionally incapable of being honest." It's foolproof marketing strategy. Anyone who pushes against 12 Steps, or questions some of its faulty logic, gets shunned from the group.

I'll admit, I have a lot of resentment built up against that program. I walk a fine line between bashing the program and telling my truth. But it's hard to tell my experience without pointing out how much harm that program has caused. Sure, for some (5% to 8%), it works. That's great. For them. I've also known too many people—I've had too many friends—who were hammered with 12 Step's one-size-fits-all approach, and now they are dead.

For a treatment center, why not go with 12 Steps? One, it's free. You pile these patients, whose insurance, whether private or state-sponsored, you're charging upwards of thousands a day. Then you drive them to some church basement. It costs them nothing, which increases their bottom line, and, again, if it doesn't work for you, it's *your* fault. Not the program. Not the treatment center. Not the staff. *Your* fault. You're "not ready" and they tell your family to kick you out until you are. It's totally ridiculous.

You don't have to look far to find countries taking a more pro-active approach. Canada has some great policies. The United States' answer to substance use disorder is punishment and separation. You're gonna go to jail, we're gonna take kids, we're gonna do this, we're gonna take that. Why not put that effort into getting housing or providing accessible, affordable physical and mental health care? Whatever that person needs to get their basic needs met. We just throw them in jail. That'll fix it! It's not fixing anything.

Before my son's mother died, she was facing legal issues, causing her horrible amounts of stress. Of course, they wanted her to quit using. Which is great, in theory. Except this had been her coping mechanism for years. What did they offer to take off some of that pressure? What positive solutions were being proposed? Nothing, except stepping on her neck and not letting her up. No one is going to deal well with that kind of pressure. When you've been using substances most of your adult life, how is stripping away that coping mechanism, however "unhealthy" it may be, helping? We're taking away your pain relief, and in its place, we're going to give you more pain, with an extra dose of anxiety!

There's that whole tough love thing, kicking them out good until they're calling for rehab or whatever. Sounds reasonable, until you realize you're taking somebody that already feels un-loved, unworthy—who feels worthless—and now you're going to separate them more, and further cement their belief that nobody cares. These people already feel like they're a piece of shit, because society has told them that since they were kids (thanks again, DARE).

There's so much work to be done. But it's not hopeless. In the few short years that I've been involved in harm reduction, I've seen *some* positive changes. It's happening, slowly, but it *is* happening. We're starting to see society wake up to the lies that they've been fed, and many are reading and researching for themselves, instead of listening to their cousin's or Uncle Bob's friend, the taxi driver.

We have a long way to go, but I think we're heading in the right direction. We're slowly seeing people turn away from the stigma and shame approach. More and more people are seeing programs such as syringe exchanges, for what it really is: a community service. People are starting to see such a service doesn't just benefit the drug user; it's helping communities reduce the HIV and hepatitis rates, and much more.

There's so much to it; there's so much more to it than what people have been lead to believe. I think people are starting to see it. Change is coming!

Mike can be reached at michael7332@gmail.com. **Never Use Alone can be reached at 877-696-1996.**

MICHAEL KELLY

Stepping out of the California Prison System, I was looking for a job. I ended up working at a sober house in San Francisco. By the late nineties I was working at a needle exchange in Hollywood, downtown Los Angeles. That is when it hit me: this is harm reduction. I am a harm reductionist—guess I always have been. It's pretty much where punk rock & Buddhism intersect. Some people look down on the term harm reductionist. Me? I've been called worse by better people.

Art has played a huge role in my harm reduction work, outreach tools, images, gallery shows. My art and collections began in the eighties. I have a poster that says, *AIDS Can Blow Your High*. This was from 1988. It was part of a big subway campaign in New York City. People were freaking out about it because there was a needle on it. And that is like a collector's item now.

For me, this visual component of harm reduction has proven invaluable. Confronting people's misperceptions have been instrumental. Disturb the comfortable, right? That's always been a huge part of my outreach, my communication—challenge the status quo and outdated modes of thinking that hinder recovery. At the same time, artwork gets around some of the trappings of the written word. Art, in many ways, is timeless. Language, because it's so concise, leaves less open to interpretation, so what was okay to say yesterday might not be okay to say tomorrow. Art is a way around that. If somebody's upset with a particular image, that's their interpretation. Often, when somebody wants to take a piece down or finds it offensive, that often means it's a great piece of art! They have the issues with it, and to defend an image, you simply say that's not what that means. Our goal in harm reduction is to assist people, help them out, and if they want it, lend a hand towards a better life. We're trying to reach people, help people, and save lives.

My harm reduction journey has been a thread of opportunities, connecting one to another. Currently, I'm managing a syringe service program, which is another new name. We used to call them needle exchanges. Now it's a syringe service program or SSP. Seems like a small name change, but one term (needle exchange) can be seen as negative i.e. "one for one", whereas the other—syringe service program which is an array of services—it normalizes getting safe supplies and helps remove stigma. It's still a battle.

I remember when we were trying to get an SSP up and running in Plymouth (MA) which was difficult. This wasn't San Francisco or Buffalo, or even a bigger Massachusetts city like Cambridge or Dorchester. We are talking Plymouth, a rural beach town, seasonal population, etc. During conversations about potentially opening this program, I was constantly urging people to look at what harm reduction means. Harm reduction is about education, community, service. We do HIV and Hep-C testing. We do Narcan distribution. And, then in the fine print, we also do needle exchange, as well as crack or meth pipes, boofing kits, safer sex supplies and support services, clothing, snacks and connection to treatment services if desired. Anything else a person needs. Because if it helps keep them comfortable or alive another day, that's a good thing.

Where I work is the result of a federal study that focused on four states: Ohio, Kentucky, New York, and Massachusetts, targeting the areas needing the most help with overdose prevention due to increased fatalities in order to get Narcan into peoples' hands. There were services in these states but they weren't consolidated. That made it harder to get the word out. That also made it tougher for someone to access benefits. In communities like this one, when you face this kind of struggle, having services spread out, life itself tends to get in the way. Around the time our program started, COVID hit. This isn't a program that works over Zoom! You need personal interaction—face to face. The idea was to get Narcan in people's hands, which isn't possible online. This was a collaborative effort of a bunch of agencies, and basically anybody who might be in contact with someone at risk of an overdose: active users, their friends, families, anyone who can administer Narcan and save lives. We had an ambitious target number, shooting for eight hundred doses in the community. And we went way beyond the study's target. Before the study ended, I personally handed out almost 1,400 kits. As a result, people started surviving overdoses more often, which provides more time—time to get educated, time to get support. As result of this effort, here in Plymouth, we now have an SSP. And we also have a new methadone clinic. That may seem like a footnote statement but it's huge! So many of us are working in conjunction; there are a lot of moving parts, significant effort by many agencies, to make this work. This is still how I split my time. I run the SSP program in the day and I am active in the art and recovering communities at night, which are wonderful spaces to be in.

At the time we were putting these programs together, I was also working in a recovery center where we incorporated a lot of harm reduction strategies. We offered alternatives to regular treatment structures, like the peer run Refuge Recovery. We also offered Reiki, yoga, and art groups plus a few different 12 Step groups. But our goal never changed. These programs were for people to get their lives together. If sobriety is part of that? Even better! Personally, I'm still a 12 Step dude that is into Buddhist teachings. It works for me. That does not mean it will for everyone. I feel comfortable straddling those two worlds. It's a great skillset to offer others. For me it's this combo is the discipline I needed. It's funny, a couple of months ago my brother called me "a social butterfly that hates everybody." I said, "That sounds poetic." I had to think about it for a day or two. Eventually it made me think about a Charles Bukowski quote (I think most people in harm reduction know his story). When Bukowski was asked, "Do you hate people?" he responded, "I don't hate them. I just feel better when they're not around." I'm sure there's a few words missing from that quote, but you get the gist. When my brother said it, though, I was offended at first. I was like, "What the hell's that even mean?" But my brother wasn't criticizing me. He was pointing out the distance I need to keep people to stay sane. He was saying, "You're in all these different camps all the time, and you're able to pull back. It's not like a real deep investment in the sense of you having to stay put wherever you are." And I got that. I think that's a great tool for someone like me to have. I'm still human. People are still people. We all aren't going to have the same points of view. And that's good.

Personally, I can struggle with folks who are strictly abstinent based. I am an artist; I am a harm reductionist—as a Buddhist, my person embodies more than just one thing. I often say recovery is about mixtures. I remember telling this to my friend Adrienne and she responded, "We mixed our drugs and alcohol. We can mix recovery up too."

I've met many drug users who've struggled with 12 Step programs or abstinence, but who still want to improve their lives. It doesn't help anyone to badmouth a certain treatment modality. Your experience is your experience. It does a disservice to be hypervigilant on campaigning for or against a certain format of recovery. At that point, people might shut down or stop trying. *I am not married to your outcome.*

I had to choose to get sober. I love, love drugs. If you can use them without negative impact, good for you. For me, personally, I can't. I don't have that off switch. Doesn't matter if it's drugs and alcohol, smoke, online shopping, buying Pumas, or sex and tattoos. Whatever it is people like me like to do; I usually can't stop. I just try to navigate towards healthier things so I am able to live in harmony with my experiences. I don't want to end up in prison, I'm not going to die (from drug use), and I am not going to ruin somebody else's life. Nobody's life is going to get ruined by my sneaker habit, though, heard?

I've been working in health care since 1996. I got sober in 2007. You can do the math. I was still able to help people and earn a living even strung out. Drug use does not automatically render someone useless. I needed the time to get healthy and be free to get across the sober line, and harm reduction is one of the tools I used. I've spent time on both coasts, but I am a Massachusetts dude at heart. Sometimes, I don't even know how I survived working in healthcare in California. Viewing life as a collage of many experiences helped. I remember we were doing this outreach program in the San Jose jail. I would go to the dorms, and I'd have some educational materials, handouts, comic books, things like that, and I tried to round up a bunch of guys to take these classes. And I knew how to talk to the prisoners. I'd shut off the TV and be like, "Hey, listen up! I'd like to talk to you." And the inmates would say, "Who's this skinny fucking guy with a Boston accent think he is?" But once we started a conversation, a dialogue, where I was treating them as equals and not talking down to them like they were used to, we'd get on great! I could tell them what we had to offer and they were able to hear that because I was speaking *with* them, not *at* them. Then these cats could see what we had going on. The classes were always well attended. These were important classes on issues like HIV and Hep-C education. I was even able to share tips on nutrition and stress reduction. I'm dating myself with this, but sometimes we could rent a couple of movies (VHS) from Blockbuster for these guys. They'd be stoked about that, to be able to catch up on current releases. But it was all an avenue to open a line of communication for me, for us, for those in the treatment and recovery community, to offer a lifeline. I knew how to move in those spaces.

For me it's always been about bridging all these different pathways, "pollenating communities" or "connecting." If someone is suffering, how can we help them out? That's what I'm about. I see a lot of suffering due to drugs and alcohol, poverty, racism, just straight hate. With substances, whether it's people who are taking drugs or it's their families, friends, or loved ones, if it's impacting folks harshly or negatively, it gets labeled with terms like "alcoholism" or "addiction" or "abuse." But it's the suffering aspect that needs to be addressed. It helps to view this through that dharma lens. This person is suffering. How can we do the outreach that Buddha and Christ and all these cool teachers did? How can we provide some non-judgmental support for this person? Sometimes, just kindness will help.

When I got into recovery, I was connected to Dharma Punks. I was connected to Buddhism. Punk rock, art freaks, the outsiders. I quit smoking before I stopped doing other drugs. I was a vegetarian doing yoga. But I was still shooting speed balls. You know what I mean? SF style. I loved the Tenderloin. Did I bottom out? I don't know. Bottoming out is under dirt, the final act, so I guess I didn't. I turned forty, and took a good, hard look at my life. I didn't like what I saw. I could continue to tread water, settling for less, living by that "I always need more" mentality, which I could not satisfy no matter what I did. Or I could make a change. Since I was already learning about Buddhism, I figured I could use the simple five precepts of Buddhism, the last of which encourages avoiding mind-altering substances. It seemed doable at that point. I had already started on the path. I thought, "Okay, I can add this to the not killing, not stealing, refraining from sexual misconduct and the gossip, the lying— refraining from drug or alcohol use was only going to help." I saw how using contributed to many of my destructive behaviors. Since I had already begun working on these other parts of me, I thought, "Why not jump in all the way?" I could use that "no off switch" to better myself. I am an "off the high board" kind of guy. I don't check to see if there's water in the pool, I just jump. I began to realize that the same approach that got me *into* trouble could be turned around and used to help get me *out* of it too. Those behaviors seem to be part of my genetic makeup, but they don't excuse my behaviors. I have two brothers. My older brother never got high, never got arrested, never tormented our family, never did all the crazy stuff. Me and my younger brother lived that junkie life. So, you have the three of us. We have the same parents. We grew up in the same house with the same rules, lessons, and moral compass. Our older brother went down one road, and we went down another. Sometimes there are life choices and sometimes there are not. As I move forward in health care, recovery, and harm reduction, I approach it as, "How can I help you? What do you need? What do you think?" I tap into Buddhist principals.

Prior to opening the SSP in Plymouth, we had a team meeting about house rules. Basic stuff: watch your language, don't blast your radio, respect, confidentiality, and safety—and the big one: no hate. I was sitting with staff and some bosses, and someone asked, "What do you think, Michael?" I said, "I just want to add one line to this, and it needs to be on the TOP: *Kindness is always the response, for staff and participants.*" And that is the number one house rule!! Kindness requires flexibility, love and tolerance of others. This is our code. You can't attach yourself to one outcome. Doing that is a dangerous way to think. It's been easy to navigate myself in this field, because I'm the same fucking dude with everybody. Whether it's the bosses and staff, the participants, my recovery platforms, my friends, family and neighbors. I must be my authentic self. And if I can do that in a non-attached, non-judgmental way, I can always help people. It's how I view life—and recovery. If I can do something to help you, I will.

We—I—need to keep learning to be okay and stay teachable. We must understand these multiple pathways. We need to be a little more hardcore and not so sensitive—feelings are become way to distracted; respect is far more useful and real.

I might be at a meeting, walking on the street or at Walmart and I can be talking to somebody about my recovery, healing or overdoses and someone will ask, "How do you do this? How do you stay sober? You don't even smoke weed!" I'm like, "I'm a junkie, nothing is ever enough. My recovery is about mixtures. I'm trying to live day-to-day while the world's on fire. Dude, drop by our harm reduction program."

Michael can be reached at mjk67@hotmail.com

ERICA POELLOT

When it came time for me to embrace harm reduction, I can say I was both a ready convert and (also) not. I am somebody who has wrestled at various times with a substance use disorder, which is how I've come to understand it. I knew little about harm reduction as an approach for healing at the time I was ready to make some changes. Out of sheer necessity, I quickly became embedded in 12 Step fellowships. In doing so, I adopted their language and understanding of what constituted "recovery," a word I have since stopped using to describe the process by which I have renegotiated my relationship with substances.

I hung out in 12 Step spaces for over fourteen years. At the same time, I was watching and hearing the stories of friends of mine who were still using and struggling to find spaces and places to connect with care, and who were contracting Hepatitis C, HIV at an alarming rate. They were overdosing, dying. Their stories resonated with me, perhaps more than the stories I was hearing inside the rooms. I increasingly began to experience 12 Step spaces as painfully exclusive and intolerant of different ways of understanding one's relationship with substances and legitimate pathways to healing. In particular, the 12 Step communities I was part of did not consider a more expansive substance use spectrum, approaches to healing that were not abstinence based, nor did they condone the use of medications for substance use disorder. I watched numerous people edged out of 12 Step communities for using medication to treat substance use disorder, having been told they were not sober. I saw others ostracized for continuing to use substances they had not used chaotically. It was hard for me to watch people being erased from these spaces.

During this time, I moved to New York and had the opportunity to connect with the National Harm Reduction Coalition. There, I was able study with Don McVinney. As part of my graduate field work, I worked with a syringe service provider that operated a handful of mobile-only units. I started accompanying staff on their runs. I remember feeling very uncomfortable with the premise of harm-reduction strategies, such as sterile syringe distribution, as it challenged what I had been taught in 12 Steps. What I had been learning about harm reduction to this point was presented in this very intellectual, theoretical, kind of scholastic/academic way. And I think that, in and of itself, that wasn't enough to convince me of the power of harm reduction.

One day we were in Brooklyn, in a neighborhood in Coney Island. I had the opportunity to sit in the van and listen in to the conversations that people were having. While there were conversations about safer injecting practices and overdose prevention and other harm reduction strategies, the heart of these conversations were stories about children and partners, connecting with one another, sharing hopes and dreams, and everyday happenings that they wanted to share. There were beautiful and enduring relationships that had been sown over time. I had the opportunity to see people find community, make connections and positive changes in their lives, which aligned with their own values. These changes were self-directed and moreover encouraged. What was most evident was that people were loved. Having the opportunity to witness the transformative potential of harm reduction community coincided with me making some personal decisions around how I understood my own use and how I wanted to pursue healing.

Having been deeply rooted in a singular way of understanding and talking about my substance use, I struggled to access language and conversation spaces with which to reimagine and recast my healing process. I found an incredible friend and thought-partner in Dr. Sharon Stancliff, who helped me tease apart the challenges and cognitive dissonance I was experiencing with 12 Step. She helped me push back against the pathologizing messages I had absorbed about my personhood and my substance use, which allowed me to see an expansive range of possibilities and pathways. Mainly, she listened, she was present, and she made space for me to grapple with all the questions I had been afraid to ask aloud. She helped me cultivate the courage to re-claim my agency, my dignity, and the ability to author my own story.

This opportunity to experience harm reduction in terms of relationship—and community-building as an act of love enabled me to look at my substance use through the lens of (shared) human experience—entirely absent of judgment. This helped me ask and answer questions, professionally and personally. To imagine how differently treatment looks when we suspend moralizing and dehumanizing language about people who use drugs. How different healing might look when you don't drag and attach dehumanizing and stigmatizing constructs to very human behaviors. This more inclusive approach allowed me to accept facets of myself I had felt immense shame about. Harm reduction, in community, helped me reclaim my voice.

My definition of harm reduction shapes my approach. For my ordination interview, I described it as an invitation into relationship, into connection, and into community. This connection, this inclusion, this invitation shaped by radical compassion and loving regard for the fullness of one another's humanity. I have experienced this as the embodiment of harm reduction, the expression of the radical welcome and worth of all stories. Harm reduction makes sacred space, inviting all—especially people who find themselves at the many margins, people who are creatively, desperately, intently and faithfully searching to find ways to carry their burdens. It makes space for people to tell their stories, to own their whole story with the wholeness of who they are. It foregrounds the wisdom and leadership of people with lived and living experience, which ensures that more people have an opportunity to see reflections of themselves in all our communities and sacred places. Harm reduction is love that stands with people. It says come as you are, you are loved, and wholly enough, holy and enough. In this way, I have come to understand harm reduction as a spiritual practice—a definition I've put into action.

For me, as a faith leader, a person of faith, I understand my relationship to the Divine, to God, in the context of my call to harm reduction ministry, and that is the call to lead with love, work for justice, and connect with compassion. Harm reduction is both an invitation to see our personal stories as part of the larger story of love and creation, as well as an opportunity to be challenged and changed by stories other than our own.

It is my prayer, that harm reduction be further embedded in the root structures of all systems, all relationships, all communities, such that equity, justice, and love grow. Harm reduction as a creative force exists in the fertile gray space between and beyond false binaries, between use and non-use, peer and professional, self and other, all the ways that we have used to disintegrate connection, to accentuate difference, and to delineate power. It is my prayer that we learn to embrace the gray, to embrace the life-giving power of harm reduction.

Harm reduction is the power to co-create narratives that enjoin all of us, each of us, in the story of love and hope.

Rev. Erica can be reached at erica@faithinharmreduction.org

TESSA REYNOLDS

Rose is my middle name. I go by Tessa Rose. It's more of an anonymous name, but that's my name on social media, so it's out there now.

I came to harm reduction by accident. I didn't really know anything about it and I was even already practicing it. When I got on my own recovery path, I was utilizing harm reduction strategies. I was learning there was a wide spectrum of healing out there, and maybe abstinence isn't for everyone; that was really helpful for me.

I went to school to get my certification in drug and alcohol studies at City College. And I remember in class, when the teacher talked about harm reduction, a lot of folks had a hard time wrapping their head around the concept, like, "Oh, wow, how could we do this?" And for me, it really just fit. I was like, Oh, I get this. It matches my recovery story more now that I understand what harm reduction is. To me, harm reduction was another avenue that gave people autonomy—letting people know it was okay to be "where they're at."

Plus, having worked in abstinence-based treatment, I think this resonated more for me. I was working in a system that wasn't helping participants as much as I saw it hurting them. You'd have people who were in the program giving positive urine tests, and it was hard to watch people being punished and exited from treatment for manifestations of their trauma. It was heartbreaking. I was truly a harm reductionist living and working in an abstinence-based world.

Approaching treatment from the angle of a harm reductionist was amazing. I could connect with people on a different level than other counselors, because it changed the power dynamic in our relationship. Participants would become empowered to have a say in what would work for them with changing their relationship with substances. I didn't care as much about drug testing. I understand that participants in a group setting might not want to admit they'd engaged in substance use over the weekend because of the stigma and shame places on drug use. I might not drug test someone because I understand the process and if they were positive they could be "exited" from the support they're receiving. My heart would see the progress folks were making and a drug test didn't always show that in the results. I didn't see the benefit of prosecuting or shaming people into changing, it just never works. I witnessed the benefit of using compassion, collaboration, and understanding as essential tools to help someone heal. What I saw happening in my groups might be different than what a test result would show an outsider like their probation officer. I had people who were "mandated" to treatment asking me if they could stay longer when they were successfully completing their program, while other counselors had people not even showing up to their groups. I knew it was something about this harm reduction approach that was giving people the dignity and power to change.

Drug diversion work started to wear on me. I had to drug test people three times because of their diversion program, mostly knowing they'd fail and be in trouble with the system. These were the exact same people who were making *great* strides in their healing and just weren't at the "total abstinent" phase yet. I never saw how kicking people out of services because they weren't abstinent yet, was actually helping people. I got into the helping field to actually help people, not hurt them because our racist drug laws say "it's wrong."

There was one specific case I will never forget. This young guy came to our program, after he was caught using and possessing heroin. He had severe scoliosis and kept using cannabis as a way to manage his chronic pain. I'm a big advocate of using alternative paths, with or without cannabis. Okay, so the rules were if you had THC in your system, the levels need to decrease during your time in the program showing you are not using. As we all know THC tends to show positive test results for up to 30 days. He understood. He was doing amazing, his life was getting better and then his final test went up like .01 mg of THC. In the eyes of the system, that is a positive result, and he was immediately discharged and excluded from treatment. How is that right? Now my job is to kick this guy out, shame him, reject him and cut off his support. Everything we've been building together is done, for one test? How can I keep doing this? The folks who need services and support the most are being told to leave, I just couldn't take part any longer. Luckily, the position I'm in now allows me to make real and lasting positive changes for people who use drugs and other marginalized communities, at the government level.

If we look at Maslow's hierarchy of need, we can see the basics— the food, the shelter, etc., but that's just the tip of the iceberg. We're bypassing a lot in traditional treatment settings by unconsciously saying, "You, meet us where we're at!" Instead of, "Let me meet *you* where *you're* at." I've always had this thing in me to just be present for them in a time of need. It's like we design these systems and protocols where you have to change prior to coming to get the services. You have to be abstinent before you've even had time to learn how to do that or even decided if you want to do that. This didn't work for me. We don't do that with other "diseases," if we're going to qualify substance use as a disease in the DSM—that's not how other folks are being treated when they're physically sick. This is the only disease we classify with consequences and then try to treat with consequences, it's nonsense.

Working in permanent supportive housing, I saw some of the most vulnerable folks in our society. We were connecting. I was helping them build something inside of themselves, helping repair damage. Even though they might be engaging in substance use, we were still making progress. It's okay to have a different perspective on substance use. One size does not fit all.

Prior to getting that job, I never noticed all the elements of harm reduction working together, like mutual aid, housing, healthcare and public health. I didn't think about how everyone in the world practices harm reduction—how it has been the primary healthcare model for the 21st century. I loved motivational interviewing—I still love motivational interviewing, which is harm reduction without the label of harm reduction, right? Teaching folks, how to connect with people, how to roll with it, how to let people have their own autonomy and set their own goals, it's everything that motivational interviewing encompasses.

I didn't come to harm reduction thinking it's abstinence or harm reduction. For me, they always belong on the same recovery continuum.

I remember when I watched an interview with Dr. Gabor Mate, he said something profound. He said, "Why would we open clinics, where people have to go behind our clinic and inject with dirty puddle water, get septicemia, abscesses and all of these chronic health conditions, when we could simply invite them in, offer them a cup of tea, give them a human connection, and sit with them and see how their day is going?"

That really hit me. I was like, "Aha! *That's* what I've been working in!" I've been working in a system where the folks who need the most help are not allowed to even enter the building. What do you think they are going to do? I'll tell you—the same thing they've been doing, but with extra guilt and shame. How does that help in recovery?

Alcohol, which is legal, can cause more damage to the human body and brain than the "bad" illegal substances. So why do we have all these "bad" drugs, but these other ones are legally sanctioned? It all comes down to class and racism. Who's perceived to use alcohol? Caucasian people, you know, European folks. So we'll keep that legal. This started making me look more into the intersections of how drug use hits certain populations and how it's then perceived and how we stigmatize it, and everything that's wrapped into that good ol' War on Drugs. You can't unsee it once you've learned racism is the answer to why heroin, cocaine/crack, cannabis, peyote, psilocybin, and mescaline are all illegal.

While I am a full-on harm reductionist, I love working with abstinence-only based programs. I want to help people like me, help them understand and use these techniques, tools, and skills we learn through harm reduction. They can help everyone. They don't just work for somebody that's unhoused. They don't just work for somebody that "doesn't want to get sober," as it's viewed in some people's eyes.

I think, since the beginning, I was a harm reductionist. I just didn't have the vocabulary. I didn't have the education to understand that's what it is. That's what I was doing and it was working.

So thank you, because when I read your book (*Kicking and Screaming*), it spoke to me, because of the way you connect harm reduction with 12 Steps. Which helped dissipate my shame. I was like, Oh, okay, I'm in recovery. Regardless of what folks believe recovery is. I get to define my own and I can see the successes I've had.

I remember in school, there was a classmate who was using methadone. Back then, it was kind of, "Oh, gosh, you know, you're not really sober right?" This was the consensus, the feedback from classmates. I'm thinking, look at this lady. She's at school, she's learning, she's paying bills, she's keeping her life together. There were so many positive outcomes from her taking methadone, why do you want to disrupt that?

Currently, I'm working with the 2SLGBTQIA+ community, which also includes folks that are unhoused. And really looking at harm reduction in aspects of Gender Affirming Care. I got this sticker that says, "Gender-affirming care is trauma-informed care." I'm like, Ha, ha, it is! That's harm reduction. Our language extends to so much more; it hits home.

When it comes to harm reduction, I've found there's not really one definition. For me, the first thing coming to mind is love. Like a language of love to be with people, unconditional positive regard. But it doesn't stop there. Because there's so many different aspects of harm reduction. We get caught up on the substance use aspect in society. A lot of folks don't really understand the social advocacy part, looking at the policies and drug laws that keep people oppressed. In this regard, when I think of harm reduction, I envision the liberation and freedom of providing equitable healthcare access to all. I'm learning more about harm reduction's history every day in my circles. It's very interesting. Like how it connects to the queer community, which stems from working with the Black Panthers back in the day.

I think we need to expand our understanding of harm reduction. For instance, I practiced harm reduction this morning by putting on sunscreen. I wore my seatbelt to work. We miss so many ways harm reduction applies to the 21st century right now. Fixating on the term by simply how it relates to "these illicit drug users" misses the point of it being a universal practice for all. I think that rhetoric is so harmful to folks. If you have diabetes, you're *supposed* to lower your sugar intake. That's harm reduction. I would like to see harm reduction implemented into every type of treatment modality. This goes back to education and what we're taught. Everyone engages in some sort of substance use. Caffeine, nicotine—or if not a substance, think about phones, right? They can be "addictive" and problematic. It's time to ditch the stigma.

I'm big on changing the narrative, especially within the queer community and the language we use around substance use. I've come to this conclusion recently. We have weaved this misinformed separation between drugs and alcohol, from what I know alcohol is a drug. Look at the opioid crisis. When someone ingests too much, we call it an overdose, right? And when we hear overdose, we're taught to think "someone took too much, they shoulda known better." There's a lot of stigma and negative connotation tied with the word, even though overdose it's defined as a lethal or toxic amount in one's system. Now look at alcohol. When someone drinks too much, we say alcohol poisoning. And when we hear poisoning our minds subconsciously think "a poisoning sounds like it happens to a victim, no one intentionally poisons themselves." We don't hear about alcohol overdoses in our country when essentially a high dose of alcohol is toxic for someone. In the end when we hear someone has "overdosed," it aims to put blame on the person using the substances and "alcohol poisoning" aims to place blame elsewhere. Sadly, the language is starting to shift now with fentanyl poisonings, but it still isn't good enough. This is being used to separate folks who are believed to have unintentionally consumed fentanyl opposed to those who are intentionally using Fentanyl. Language is so powerful and is used to separate us or connect us, we need to be connected. It's our human nature.

For centuries, we've used languages that perpetuate this divide. We must approach abstinence and harm reduction as part of the same continuum, like anything—like sexuality, like gender expression, like any of the things we're dissecting and looking into for answers. For instance we are fine with "bars," but not safe-consumption sites. Why? Because our language around drug use is separating and divisive. Bars are okay and safe consumption sites are bad? Even though bars are safe consumption sites. If you're in a bar, drink too much and I'm bartending, I'm gonna cut you off. If you pass out and aren't responding, I will call an ambulance for you. I'm doing harm reduction work at a bar even if I'm not aware. Why are we treating alcohol poisonings differently than drug overdoses? It's *all* poisoning right?

I'm a certified addiction treatment counselor, but it's such a binary language, addicted or non-addicted. We know that's not how people actually use substances. I switched to saying "chaotic use" to help better describe people's relationship with substances. I was in a stage of chaotic use, someone's using chaotically, which is problematic, so that's what is addressed. The high risk behaviors rather than an absolute, humans are complex and so are our relationships with substances.

Carl Hart said in his new book, "Take the harm out of harm reduction, because when we say harm reduction, subconsciously, we are connecting all substance use with harm." I'd never thought about it that way, but it makes sense.

I'm not looking to change who people are. I'm trying to help people work through the trauma they've endured from simply existing. Let's stop stigmatizing each other. Let's not keep each other down because you believe may not be what's best for someone else. The person that knows what's best for them is the person living in their own life.

Tessa can be reached through deedeestoutconsulting@gmail.com

JESS TILLEY

Harm reduction, literally, saved my life. I come from a working class family. By the time I was fifteen, I was looking for something that could help me be present without having to be present. The first time I did heroin, that was it; I was able to be around people. I remember thinking *heroin* saved my life. I was in tenth grade, in one of those programs for gifted students, and I remember looking around my classroom of seventeen people, thinking I don't think anyone else did heroin on their spring vacation. And that shame and guilt I felt.

A friend who was very important in my life had what we referred to at the time as full-blown AIDS, and they were involved in activism. I learned about ACT UP and I had been to different rallies. I was getting involved very young. So I knew what harm reduction was. I was thirteen the first time I saw a Four H shirt. I laugh at the language, because wearing a Four H shirt now would get you cancelled. (Back then 4 H stood for heroin addicts, homosexuals, Haitians, and hemophiliacs!)

I moved to Northampton, Massachusetts, when I was nineteen.

I'd grown up with a very tight knit group of friends. Two of my best friends were using and injecting by age sixteen. I used to think, "Oh my God, how can I help them?" There were no programs, no resources for people, especially young queer women. Little did I know that within three years, I would be in the same position.

I experienced something pretty traumatic. By the end of my teen years, I knew that feeling. I knew heroin would take me back to that safe feeling. What I couldn't understand was the chaos that would almost kill me. I used dangerously. I had track marks, I was wearing long sleeves in the summertime, and I was one hundred twenty-seven pounds, which was really skinny for me. They told me about a needle exchange program, and it took me almost two weeks to go. In those days, we didn't have syringe access, pharmacy access. That wouldn't come for like another ten years. Like I said, my use was reckless. I know it's where I got Hep C, sharing a syringe, and I had a really bad abscess. When I went to needle exchange, I lied, like people do. I said I was "seeking help," because we're taught by the system to lie.

Through tears, I claimed to "have a friend who's using and I don't know how to help them." Monique Tula was a health educator at Tapestry Needle Exchange (Adam Butler was also there). They told me something along the lines of, "You don't have to do that here." It was like I could finally be *me*. And I remember they looked me in the eye as they said it. Two things happened that day. One, I realized nobody had looked me in the eye and talked to me with dignity, compassion, and respect before, and two, that it came from a place of absolute honesty. They shot straight from the hip. Here's what's going on with your body and here's what we can do to help you. Here are the tools. And I remember the word "tools." That made sense to me. The second thing I realized that day: I got hit by this harm reduction philosophy, and I wanted what these people had. (Does that sound familiar?)

The 12 Steps presented some, let's say, challenges. I was queer. I was a woman, I was poor, and I came from the working class. There were already so many, quote, unquote, strikes against me. I had been arrested by that point. I kept hearing I was a bad person. They said I was a failure, morally. I knew that wasn't true. Some people pushed back and insisted harm reduction gave me an excuse. No, it gave me a reason to live! I saw people using harm reduction to make their lives better, and I wanted that, too. People in harm reduction didn't run from who they were—they embraced it and were very open about their life experience. So I kept coming back, and hanging around, until one day someone asked, "Do you want to volunteer?" And they paid you cash to do it!

This was before the second ever Harm Reduction Coalition Conference. I wasn't gonna go. I didn't realize there were other people doing this work. For me, Northampton was the be- all-end-all of harm reduction. We were part of this phenomenal community. I went to the conference, which was a year or so after I first started going into the exchange; it blew my world wide open. Back then the conference had maybe one hundred fifty people. They were panels, like, "How to Make Your Own Opium" and, and another was for drug-user organizing. This phenomenal queer woman of color ran it. I'd found my family.

It's important to note: my use didn't stop. I don't want people to assume, as many have, that I stopped all drug use. I did not.

But as I got more connected, I felt like I had a purpose, and *from there* my use became less problematic. My relationship to drugs—and more importantly myself—changed. I started to learn how to be in my own skin. Obviously, I had years of therapy too. We can't discount the shame.

That was another by-product from that first day at needle exchange. I'd had such shame connected to my trauma, and it was just piled on. Nobody should carry that much shame, especially so young. I was mired in it. By learning to accept who I was and where I came from, it went away, that shame. I wish I could say it *stayed* gone (shame has a way of coming around again). For a brief moment in that room, with somebody handing me a little brown bag full of supplies, I suddenly felt whole. That was probably the first time in my life that I can recall where I didn't feel shameful.

In many ways, being part of that community did for me the same thing heroin had. Except this was healthy. It wasn't replacing one substance for another. This was how people are supposed to be in community with one another. If people were really like this with people, there would be less need for heroin. I hope this book will show that harm reduction is a culture. It's more than a set of tools. That's part of it. But to me, it reminds me of motivational interviewing. It is a way of being with people. And then there's the strategies and skills that go under that. But first, you got to really give a shit, really love the people that you're working with.

Some of the best harm reductionists I know never used drugs. My first time sitting in a motivational interviewing training, I said this was a daily practice with a set of tools I'd been given.

Because of the way the drug war trains our brain, I doubted myself and my progress. There was a point when I left harm reduction to go back to AA, and I was miserable—so miserable—I was hateful and angry. Everything came out the side of my neck. On paper, I looked great. I was buying a house. I was working in a nursing home. I was engaged to a guy. I woke up one morning in New Jersey, in a house I loved, and said, I can't do this anymore. I went and applied at the Cambridge Needle Exchange, and I got the job. I didn't look back. I gave up my house, gave up everything. I came back to harm reduction. And, you know, I realized I never really left. It was the feeling of coming home and I vowed to stay. Yeah, so they'll have to drag me away kicking and screaming.

When people ask me to define "harm reduction," it's tricky to put in context. We didn't have terms like "radical love" or "radical acceptance" back in '96. Harm reduction extends beyond tools and principles.

It's a community. Harm reduction is simplicity. It's what we are supposed to do as human beings, when we say love one another. I don't mean to say, "God's love," but when I think about what God is to *me*—I was raised to believe as a Catholic—*that* is the spirit of harm reduction.

Mark Kinsley shared this with me many times over the years. He called us "the rag pickers of humanity." Rag pickers go out every day and they search for things of value, the things that other people consider trash but we find beauty in them. We find those who have been cast away by society, unwanted, unloved, unneeded. We shine them up and we bring them back to the fold. Mark once said to me, "There's nothing like watching the light come back in somebody's eyes." Sometimes that light is

211

so easy to ignite just by listening and seeing somebody. For me, harm reduction is being seen, with our scars and our mess, our blood and our tears, and also our beauty.

I have a little problem called being an overachiever. Harm reduction allowed for me to make mistakes, and to learn from them. And I think about my mentors—they didn't have a generation before them to look to. They were just free-falling, flying by the seat of their pants. I realized harm reduction allowed me to make mistakes so that the next generation didn't have to make them. I'm so thankful for the mistakes I made. Some were small. Others were a little bigger. But there's always forgiveness. Harm reduction *is* forgiveness. That's something I have to remember when I'm being really hard on myself.

I was watching some video online. And they said we have to learn to work with people that we may not necessarily like. I think where we are in harm reduction, we are at a very crucial point. If you had told me twenty—even ten—years ago that harm reduction would be a household phrase, I would have laughed. At that time, we were fighting so hard, just to have public health accept us.

I don't want to see people that distribute Naloxone call themselves a harm reductionist, because that alone is not harm reduction. If you're giving out Naloxone, but you're judging the person you're giving it to, you need to step out and re-evaluate who you are, and what you are doing. I want to see harm reduction fully embraced. But also, we need to have the humility to be able to step back to teach and let new leaders emerge. I think there is an attitude that we were here first; it's our way or no way. I came in on the tail end of the first generation. We have to realize that things are changing. There's a ton of money

212

coming and there will be organizations and agencies that hated us and still hate us. We can't change that, but what we *can* do is work beside them, to educate and better understand. We don't have to work with them, but we have to work *beside* these organizations and use honest dialogue to teach. We wouldn't be here had we not been taught by the first generation.

Sometimes we can argue over what constitutes progress. We have this inward firing squad mentality, cancel culture, etc. We're only hurting one another. I don't want to see black and brown individuals continuously dying of fatal overdoses and having harm reduction programs claim that overdose rates are dropping. There has to be a shift in classism and racism around harm reduction. I believe that the powers that work against us are trying to set up this divisive atmosphere.

I was interviewing people for the Massachusetts Oral History Project. People of all backgrounds were saying that the story perpetuated is how harm reduction was started by straight white men in suits. That isn't true. In sticking to that narrative, we're undoing all the hard work and erasing the identity of the strong, black queer women who started this movement. We have to preserve our history. That's paramount if we are to move forward.

I'm going to go back to what I said earlier, that you do not have to be a person who has lived experience to be a part of harm reduction. That thinking belongs to the past. We have living experience, which is in the present.

Harm reduction is not enabling. We're helping folks survive another day. I think it becomes cliquey and ego-driven when we insist a person needs to have used drugs in order to be a harm reductionist. Or you have to have been someone who traded sex. That does not give you an entry into declaring yourself a harm reductionist. You can be an amazing harm reductionist who never used. It's about your heart. Harm reduction is heart, soul, and caring for one another.

Jess can be reached at jtilley@hrh413.org

PART 3

TREATMENT – HARM REDUCTION
COUNSELORS/THERAPISTS/
RESEARCHERS

KENNETH ANDERSON

I will take you on a journey. It's a crooked one. My path to harm reduction has been anything but straight. For me, harm reduction is, in the words of the late Dan Bigg, "Any positive change."

I grew up on a farm in the middle of nowhere about 40 miles west of Eau Claire, Wisconsin. I lived there until I was twenty and started college in Eau Claire. I'm actually a high school dropout, because they were teaching me nothing in school, so I dropped out to read Kant and teach myself calculus. In Eau Claire, where I went to college, there's no drugs except pot, or if there is, it just wasn't around me. I tried cocaine exactly once; the only time I ever saw it. I've never seen heroin, LSD, etc. After a year as an undergrad at Eau Claire, I went as a foreign exchange student to Japan and wound up spending six years there, teaching myself Classical Japanese, Classical Chinese, and Japanese dialectology. Eventually, I returned to the US and wound up in a master's program in linguistics at the University of Minnesota in Minneapolis.

In the mid-1990s, while I was finishing my master's, I started working as a shelver at the public library. I had started drinking heavily while in Japan to deal with depression and insomnia. I completed my master's in linguistics, but the government had fouled up my financial aid so that I had no way to fund a PhD, so I went from part time to full time at the public library.

I loved working at the public library because it's such a purely socialist organization, and because I spent most of my time in the closed stacks with all these great old books, many of which weren't even cataloged so people didn't know they existed. I also loved listening to pre-war blues and drinking heavily when I was off from work. I figured it didn't matter so long as I did a better job than anyone else there. I always figured that I was sleeping it off, and didn't realize there could still be alcohol in my system eight hours later. However, my boss cared more about whether I drank than the quality of my work, and eventually I got fired. I found myself homeless and went to the county for help.

I made a request for chemical-free housing, but also said please don't give me anything to do with the 12 Steps because those meetings make me want to drink! When I said that, the county worker blew a gasket. He told me, "You're sicker than anyone else I know. I am going to send you to the drunk house as a punishment until you accept that AA is the one true way." So they sent me to a wet house, effectively saying, "Drink yourself to death; you're hopeless."

Of course, AA isn't the only way. If you look at the data from the National Epidemiological Survey on Alcohol and Related Conditions (NESARC), you see that of the 90% of people who recover from alcohol use disorder, only 10% join any sobriety organization. Most people just wake up one day and say, I'm goddamn sick of what I'm doing. And I'm gonna change. I'm gonna cut back or I'm gonna quit. And they do. And those people are not easy to locate. They don't run around saying, "I'm an alcoholic, or I used to be a drunk." They just learn they have the capability to change. That's one issue I have with Alcoholics Anonymous—this idea of powerlessness. I found the notion of "powerlessness" to be extremely toxic and harmful. For me what helps is saying, "I am not powerless! Alcohol is powerless. Alcohol is an inanimate object. It can't do anything. Alcohol can't jump off the shelf. It can't pour itself into my mouth. It has zero power. Humans are powerful by nature. They can do things. They can manipulate objects. They can choose to drink or not drink. Humans have power. Inanimate objects, like rocks or alcohol or doorknobs, have no power!"

While I was living in the wet house, I started working as the online coordinator for a group named Moderation Management. Sadly, the story everyone knows about Moderation Management and its founder Audrey Kishline isn't accurate. I remember the first meeting I had with Audrey in Minneapolis in 1996, when I was still working on my master's degree and had decided to cut back a lot on drinking so that I could finish my thesis. I told Audrey that my plan was to drink a fifth of whiskey one day a week and abstain the other six. And she said, "That's not moderation." And I said, "Yeah, but it's better than drinking a fifth four days a week." Ultimately, she reluctantly agreed.

People always talk about how the founder of MM killed four people while driving drunk, but they leave out the part that at the time Audrey had left MM and joined Alcoholics Anonymous. When she resigned from Moderation Management, she confessed in a letter that she had been going over the limits for years and lying about it. She wrote, "So I'm leaving MM to join

AA." You saw how well that worked out. Four months later, she killed two people driving drunk.

I think it's unfortunate that Audrey never understood harm reduction. Her black-and-white beliefs centered around an unattainable goal: you had to be perfect in moderation or perfect in abstinence. There was no room for imperfection in her thought process. Yet not a single newspaper ran a headline saying Alcoholics Anonymous member Audrey Kishline kills people. It was all about how moderation couldn't work.

If alcohol is more powerful than humans, humans cannot stop drinking, right? Obviously, it's gonna be completely impossible. Which, of course, is Bill Wilson's big trick to make you believe in God. Because if you don't believe in God, you will drink yourself to death. Well, obviously, I didn't believe in any supernatural beings; my subconscious did not buy into that. I did try AA, but after attending meetings for a couple of months, I drank more than I ever had in my life. I drank five liters of whiskey in five days. I was in such a state of withdrawal that I had to check in to county detox, so that I didn't die from withdrawal. That's when I realized that I had to stop going to AA meetings or I would die. They would kill me.

I lived at the St. Paul wet house for two years--the whole time I was successful with my plan to abstain six days per week and drink a fifth on the seventh. My roommate was a Quaker, and I was a socialist, so we got along great because we believed the same things. While there, I'd commute every day to the public library in Edina. That's an hour bus ride from where I lived in St. Paul. Edina is a well-off suburb of Minneapolis—they have a great public library, with all these computers, whose slots were never full. Each day, I'd find all these terminals standing empty. This allowed me to be online eight hours a day, messaging with people in the online Moderation Management group.

Eventually, the online Moderation Management group decided they wanted me to be their online coordinator. And they actually paid for me to take a visit to New York City. While visiting New York, I told one of the directors about my plan to abstain six days per week and drink a fifth on the seventh, and he replied, "That might not be moderation, but it's pure harm reduction." I really hadn't heard the term harm reduction before this, but I started to investigate it now. I started volunteering at Access Works, the Minneapolis needle exchange, and this was the most transformative experience of my life. I was HOME. These were MY people. After this I breathed, ate, and slept harm reduction! I introduced all the harm reduction concepts I learned at the exchange into the online Moderation Management group, and many people ate them up. But others did not.

In 2004, I found employment and escaped the wet house, and in 2006, I moved to New York City. In the summer of 2006, Moderation Management got a new executive director, and we harm reduction folks were told we were no longer welcome. We were told that everyone in Moderation Management had to either be perfectly moderate drinkers according to Moderation Management's moderate drinking guidelines or get out. We got out and formed our own online alcohol harm reduction group, the first of its kind.

We combined the "H" in "harm reduction" with the "A" in "abstinence" with the "M" in "moderation" with the "S" in "support" and called ourselves HAMS. Our members decided to call themselves "Hamsters." In fact, we use the hamster as our mascot. So we are all hamsters. We are based on the same harm reduction principles as needle exchange programs, and we support every positive change, no matter how small.

In August of 2007, we incorporated and sent off to the IRS for the 501 (c) 3. Amazingly, we got approved in like a month. Wow. Because they say this usually takes six months to a year or more. They must have just looked at our bylaws and said these people are never gonna make any money, ever. We don't have to worry.

These days, we call Facebook home. Some people don't have Facebook accounts, so they can also sign up for the forum instead. That's the two active online support groups we have going right now. We're not doing any live meetings currently. The Facebook group and the forum each have about 12,000 members. While I was in New York City, I managed to get my financial aid straightened out and completed a master's degree in psychology and substance abuse at the New School for Social Research.

One of the fundamental principles of HAMS is that everyone is different. Everybody's thoughts work differently. You know, I can't impose what I think on anybody else. If you want to believe in god, go ahead! It's a free country. We have freedom of religion here. So, believe whatever you want to believe.

These days I'm far more accepting of AA. If it works for you? Great! You don't have to think the same way that I think, you can do it anyway you like, and of course, it's happened in the HAMS group on Facebook, too, because we have people saying, "Well, I'm moderating, but I do find that going to AA meetings is helpful to me." That might not work for me. But, hey, if it works for them? Do whatever is helpful for you. If a person wants to change, that's the question he or she will need to ask: What's working for them? Because you don't have to think the way I think. You don't have to believe what I believe. But if we're talking harm reduction, we share a common goal: what steps can we take to help make a better life for ourselves?

I quit drinking in public ages ago. Well, I do it occasionally. But I'm so moderate—I have such strict limits—if I ever drink socially, it's like no effect of alcohol at all. I will do it when in the situation calls for it. I think my last social drinking occasion was about two years ago. I much prefer to drink alone. On my weekly drinking day, I buy a fifth of whiskey, and when it's gone, I go to sleep. I drink and watch movies or listen to music, safely at home. And you know, when my booze is gone? I don't keep any in the house. So when it's gone, it's time to go to sleep.

Yeah, that's it. And nobody gets hurt. Nobody gets harmed. Except maybe the people in the movies.

Ken can be reached at hamshrn@gmail.com
https://hams.cc

PHILIP BAKER (alias)

I came to harm reduction kind of through the side door. I started my career as a California certified drug and alcohol counselor with the Department of Public Health in the horribly named Offender Treatment Program. I wound up working for them for many years. Eventually I ended up working at the Community Assessment and Services Center, which is around the corner from 850 Bryant. It's a probation building. My job was as a counselor working with probation clients for an agency called Leaders and Community Alternatives. My direct supervisor was an ex-cop who was kind of a jerk, and we clashed a lot. One day he decided to bring the metal detectors from upstairs where the probation officers were down to our clinical setting. And I told him I thought that was a really dumb idea and we shouldn't do that, and if we do, we're going to see our numbers drop—probationers aren't going to come into counseling if they're made to feel like they're back in jail, going through these metal detectors. And sure enough, he brought it down, and our numbers dropped. And I was like, "Man, I told you that was gonna happen." We were serving a traumatized group of people—traumatized by law enforcement and the criminal justice system and the metal detector was a reminder of all that. I went through some pretty difficult clashes with that agency. I decided to keep my ears open for something else. As it happened, a job came my way that changed my life.

I had a friend named Bill that worked over at Glide Harm Reduction. He called me up one day and was like, "Dude, this place is rad! We're doing good stuff here. You should come join us." I gave it a shot and I applied and got the job. I left the traditional AOD world and I went to harm reduction, and pretty quickly fell in love. You know, harm reduction is an amazing intervention. I especially like the approach towards people, and that's how I ended up in harm reduction. I've been a hardcore harm reductionist ever since. Right now, I work a full-time job in the clinical world in management where I oversee staff in a residential treatment program and withdrawal management program. But on the side, I do outreach on Wednesday nights, after hours outreach in the Tenderloin, and I work for Homeless Youth Alliance on Friday nights, where I do a bunch of harm reduction outreach stuff, just out of the sheer joy of it on my off times. I love all the people I get to be with. I'm solidly in the harm reduction world.

I'm not sure if we all mean the same thing when we say "harm reduction," you know? The way that I've come to see it over the years of doing harm reduction is two-fold. This two-fold way is straight from Eliza Wheeler, co-director of the Remedy Alliance/For the People program. Eliza talks about harm reduction being both the lowercase "harm reduction" and the uppercase "Harm Reduction." I see lowercase "harm reduction" as the *stuff* of harm reduction—the supplies, medications like suboxone and methadone, the paraphernalia of helping people make safer decisions around their drug use. You could call it the "nuts and bolts" of harm reduction. Then there's the upper-case Harm Reduction, which has a center to it which I really love and that's the philosophies of harm reduction, like *meeting people where they're at,* that sort of thing. When I go out on Wednesday or Thursday nights in the Tenderloin, in the dual problems of mass homelessness and drug use and people see me with harm reduction supplies, there's a sort of "Jedi mind trick" that's so cool because people automatically know that you're not judging them for their drug use; you're bringing supplies so that they can use safer. It's this quick therapeutic alliance that happens when you're out there doing harm reduction work, because people immediately know that you're not passing judgment on them for wherever they're at right now. I love harm reduction in that aspect—it's immediately aligning with people, and people immediately give you some trust back that they wouldn't normally give in a clinical setting, in some cold clinical environment. To me that is the sort of beauty of harm reduction. There's also the philosophical implications of honoring people's autonomy and other concepts that were life changing to me—to see how a humanistic approach to client work was so much more compassionate and more conducive to helping individuals make decisions about their lives in a way that's not judgmental.

The clinical world of substance use disorder treatment seems to have moved away from that humanistic approach over the years, and I feel like they're having a collective realization about it. I was just down at the Substance Use Disorder Conference in Long Beach put on by the State Department of Healthcare Services, and probably half the panels were about how we need to approach the 95% of people who don't even seek treatment. It seems the industry is finally looking at the shortfalls of the way we've been doing things. Here in San Francisco, we're one of the first big cities to declare itself a harm reduction city and it's been "two steps forward, one step back" lately. We did manage to get medically assisted treatment in residential settings, and I remember the pushback against that. It was really vehement. We were hearing things like, "I don't want people nodding out in my groups." There's another group of people who redo their whole website to make it sound more harm reductionistic because there's money to be had—any nonprofit organization that rebrands itself as a harm reduction agency is going to capture more dollars. It makes sense. They're chasing the dollars. A few years ago, trauma-informed care was the buzzword. Too many people throw around the latest buzzwords because doing so helps ensure that they get the funding to continue. They're going to use whatever tactic they need to put on the right face needed to find funding, but few are willing or interested in embracing the philosophies of harm reduction.

This makes me wish that people understood harm reduction better. In my current role, the conversation that I have over and over and over again with people is about having a compassionate response to individuals, and that conversation needs to happen over and over again. It makes me realize that what people don't understand about harm reduction until they fully try it, embrace it and roll it out, is that the agency will get better outcomes with compassion than fighting with people. I've learned that if I clash with the people I'm working with, I'm making my job harder because people get further entrenched in their belief system when you clash with them, or you finger wag, or whatever. It makes your job harder. Think about it. If you have a conversation with someone that you disagree with politically and come at that person with vitriol and anger and conflict, you're actually further entrenching them in their position. We see it here every day. It seems that people don't quite realize that in this work, you catch more flies with honey! It seems like that's a hard concept for people to try because basically the whole field is so moralistic. Harm reduction compassionately engaging drug users is not a moral issue—it's an approach issue. We have the evidence for this too if you go and do a little research, you can see the things that Carl Rogers was doing, the things that tons of individuals were doing back in the '50s and '60s. You can see the evidence in the moment when the clinician or Dr. Rogers is really listening to the people they're working with. I remember back when I was at City College, and I was asked to look at videos of Carl Rogers interacting with clients. I was so moved by what he was doing—or not doing. Those interactions really stood out to me because I was used to getting critiqued by certain supervisors when I was first in the field for being too client centered. I was told that I had to keep my clients at arms-length and I just wanted to know what I could do for this person and advocate for them. Now I know that this was happening because I hadn't yet found harm reduction. And harm reduction is this modality that was literally a grassroots intervention, by and for drug users, devoid of DSM-5 diagnosis clinical stuff that was developed to help clients—not clinicians. I would hope that people would really understand human nature and understand that people change in relationships. They also change in conflict but that's not often a positive change. Like I said earlier, they tend to further entrench themselves in whatever position they're in when in conflict. Whereas, if you ask open ended questions and do affirmations, all the tools that we learn through Motivational Interviewing, or some other modality based in compassion and respect, then you *can* get a positive response when you ask, "May I give you a piece of advice?" These kinds of conversations empower people to have the courage to make the changes internally themselves rather than it being instituted from the outside. I learned this over and over when I was working with people caught up in the criminal justice system and that offender treatment program, because that program was coercive as most are in criminal justice environments, labeling people "the offender" and such. I was *horrified* by that as well as, drawn to it because I am a person who came through the criminal justice system.

The first reason I went to rehab was because it was court-mandated, and the choice was drug rehab or jail. I was so sick of jail that I picked what seemed like the "easier softer way" and went to rehab. Even though I'm like the poster child for court-ordered rehab because I've been in recovery ever since, I do *not* advocate that in any way, shape, or form. I do not think that people should be mandated to treatment. Sadly, more and more people are trying to do conservatorships and forced treatment in order to respond to the open-air drug use and mass homelessness situation but we know it rarely helps long term—and in fact it causes trauma. I think it's absolutely the wrong road to go down. What we need is to do more harm reduction—fully funded and supported because the homeless situation is the worst I've ever seen it, and I've lived here my whole life.

What do I mean by funding and supporting harm reduction services? I mean that for harm reduction to make a real difference here or anywhere, it needs to be embraced, funded, brought out of the shadows, and researched. There's so much we can learn from harm reduction. San Francisco is a great model for this, because we're known as a harm reduction city. Not only did we declare that as I mentioned but we have some of the legacy harm reduction programs like San Francisco AIDS Foundation and Glide and the San Francisco Drug Users Union and more. All these places that have been built up and fully funded and they work. But at the same time, if you're a harm reduction program that gets money from the City, you're still under the watchful eye of political operatives that can yank your funding at any time and restrict what you can do. The most recent example is 1380 Howard Street's pharmacy on the first floor of the main San Francisco Department of Public Health building. There's a pharmacy there that mainly gives out Suboxone and people get referred there from all over the City. And right upstairs on the second floor is the COPE office based opiate treatment clinic, which is basically a suboxone clinic. Staff would send the prescription down to the first floor, and the pharmacy would give out all sorts of harm reduction supplies for obvious reasons. But the current mayor, London Breed, decided that she didn't want harm reduction supplies to be given out in Department of Public Health settings and yanked it all.

Sadly, the mayor also got on stage a few months ago and basically said that the open-air drug market is the fault of harm reduction services. It's not. Drugs have been bought and sold in the Tenderloin my whole life here. One of the most important things about harm reduction is that it's a pragmatic, life-saving, severely life-affirming intervention that desperately needs funding and respect. I sometimes wonder if we need to use a new way of describing harm reduction especially in San Francisco because the words "harm reduction" have become a bad word. I don't know what that is, but it feels like we need to change something. Like I said, it's "two steps forward and sometimes three back" here some days—but we all keep going because we know it's still the best way to serve drug users and they all deserve to be served and treated well.

MICHAEL CLARK

My name is Michael Clark. I'm the director for the Center for Strength-Based Strategies, which is a training and technical assistance group located in Michigan.

Harm reduction was part of my initial entry into the helping professions back in the eighties. I'd left Michigan State University and started working for a juvenile court as a probation officer and later as an abuse and neglect worker. And when you start to look at substance use dependency, and what we call "addiction treatment," back then—harm reduction made sense—and still does. For courts, it was a round peg/square hole situation because everything was abstinence-based; and yet the term harm reduction kept coming up over and over.

My harm reduction sensibilities really sharpened during the Oxy-Contin and fentanyl crisis. There was such a push back for using medications for opioid use disorder. They use the acronym MAT, which is the acronym for "Medication Assisted Treatment." This epidemic got so bad that, at one point, I was asked to do the keynote for the New York Association of Treatment Court Professionals in 2020. Literally the week before the world shut down from Covid!

The title for my keynote was "The Fight for the Soul of Treatment." I talked about treatment and I talked about the issue of harm reduction. Probably without really using the term "harm reduction." What I said was that everybody needed a seat at that table. It's amazing. You can give a keynote in front of several hundred people and not hear anything other than a "thank you" and "good job" as you finish—from the person who facilitated your keynote. But this one was different. People were emailing me and contacting me for months afterwards. Just because of the issue of having medication-assisted treatment to save lives—but not using it. The divisions were so strong. People who said those who believed in abstinence-only were called "Flat Earthers." Others who supported MAT were called greedy shills for Big Pharma. C'mon!

My take was that everybody needs a seat at *this* table. That's the proper response to a crisis. Literally. It's post-traumatic stress, right? What is something that you can't respond to? You don't have any defenses for? Our field wasn't prepared for this OxyContin and fentanyl crisis. We had to get out of our boxes.

When I was first training, I was part of the early faculty for drug courts. I was helping to develop drug courts in '99 – '02. I remember a visit to a new program. A defendant had come into the drug court with and initial urine drug-screen that held five different substances. After three months of work, he was down to just marijuana. Many rejoiced. But the prosecutor? The prosecutor on this drug court team still wanted to file a charge! And we had to sit him down and say, "This is a drug court. We're making progress!" What a fight with a stubborn legal mindset. "He's got marijuana in his system. No, he's gotta pay!" We turned this prosecutor around—but it wasn't easy.

Funny to think about it these days, when you can walk into a store down the block in Michigan and buy marijuana legally. Obviously, back then, marijuana was illegal and that's what we were up against. Culture and ethics change.

There was another situation I remember. I had just graduated with an MSW (Masters in Social Work), and I was working with a doctor, a physician, who was running a pain clinic. And there was an alcoholic who had created his own recovery program, where he only drank once a year when he went to Vegas. And I remember the doctor being upset with him, letting them know that this decision probably wasn't the best thing to do. And I remember the look on the man's face. I was doing a practicum and internship. I wasn't in a place where I could say anything. But the hurt on the man's face. He had found a really healthy place for him to be, a solution to a *huge* problem, only to be attacked and criticized by his doctor for not "doing it right." When the man left, I told the doctor what I thought. The man was engaging in harm reduction. I didn't use those words, but that's what it was. And it had been successful for him. I said we should probably be more client-centered. Of course the doctor took umbrage to that. But it was antiquated attitudes like that that helped shape my harm-reduction philosophies.

In the last few years, there has definitely been more interest in what harm reduction is. I'm at a point where I realize that a four-year undergraduate and a graduate degree did not prepare me for the field. There was such a focus on the drugs and alcohol and not nearly enough about human motivation or the process of change and how difficult it is—and how to help change occur. How in the world could the university have sent me into human services, without those two key points? How could I not know what raised or lowered motivation? How could I not know the complicated processes involved in changing behaviors and habits?

There are certainly instances where change is instantaneous. Significant life events, births, deaths, marriages, divorces, getting a job, losing a job. However, the bulk of change is a process. I was never taught what that process is, or even that a process existed. What? Importance to change and confidence that you *can* change are paramount. If you don't have both, how do you even start to take those first steps? Punishing doesn't work—we've tried that forever.

I understand evidence-based work. I personally see the merit. We also need to discuss *client*-centered work. When you start looking at this issue of ambivalence, which is a key issue for motivational interviewing, the quickest way to hijack and push the person farther away from changing (when ambivalent) is being too direct with advice and confrontation. The model originators, Bill Miller and Steve Rollnick, call this the "Fixing Reflex," which is a natural human proclivity to get in there and stop the harm. Okay, but having said that, you can literally increase their stubbornness by advocating for something they're not ready to hear. I don't want to do that anymore. I don't have time to argue. When I started, I could get people arguing with me right from the start. I didn't know any better then. I do now. There's a sense of responsibility in me. And I think this is another reason for embracing harm reduction. Once you truly understand human motivation, you understand that most people are ambivalent about poor health behaviors. Trouble is, we can't solve ambivalence with war stories, scare tactics, or punishment. If you push on one side of the ambivalence see-saw, the person will almost always push back. We know that kind of pushing is destined to fail. Why repeat it?

I was one of the first ones here in the United States to publish articles on the Strengths perspective in both juvenile justice and criminal justice. In 1997, the American Correctional Association brought their Congress of Corrections to Detroit. And out of 132 workshops, my workshop on strength-based practice was the only one that could be construed as having anything positive—anything even close to being client-centered. It was during one of these sessions, I reiterated one of the great tenants of strength-based practice, which is people have an innate sense of what's good for them. And it's our job not to install it, but rather to help bring it out, work it out. Evoke it.

When you truly understand how important it is for a client to be directly involved in his/her treatment, this absolutely has to put harm reduction back on the table. This view that only complete and utter abstinence constitutes success is nonsense. Worse, it's counterproductive. And if it's not the client's choice and they do it just to yield to authority, ultimately, it's downright detrimental to the client.

I have flown over a million miles, most of them domestically here in the United States. A trip from Boston to Los Angeles is about three thousand miles. That means I've spent almost twenty years in the air! I've encountered so many people who tout evidence showing how only total sobriety works, and because they knew however many people who had come into a program, kicking and screaming against abstinence, embraced it, embraced the 12 Steps, and look at them now! And I'm happy to see the success. But at the same time, its selective bias. Because AA or any other intervention or treatment that only recognizes total and complete abstinence sets up a "this or nothing" decision. We need options. Choices. Alternatives.

Which is why harm reduction *needs* to be part of the complement to the services that we offer. It's *that* important of an issue. The Chief Operating Officer of the National Association of Drug Court Professionals just facilitated a webinar featuring harm reduction. I was glad for that.

Again, we're seeing how important harm reduction is in terms of the current fentanyl and oxycodone crisis. A couple years ago, I was talking to frontline first responders going out to city parks and subways, shooting houses, and trying to use *some kind* of harm reduction to lower risks and help keep people alive. My center in Michigan is very focused on this idea of what happens when two people sit down in a room to talk—what happens to increase favorable outcomes? What I'm finding is that many people were not trained in how to use that first five minutes to the best of their ability—because you're not necessarily going to get more time with someone. So what do you do with that limited time? How can you maximize your efforts to help drug users to the best of your ability? The new opioid drug courts aren't always interested in traditional treatment, they want to triage people *to keep them alive.*

For me, the more options we have to save lives, the better. I can say that even though I, personally, I favor abstinence. Yet, if I'm working with someone else, that idea has to take a back seat. My personal opinion can't be part of that session. We have to consider the perspectives of our clients, first and foremost. There's too much research on how the client is the real engine to change. All change is self-change. Even if we help someone get sober, that's *guided* self-change.

Trying to scare a user by saying, "If you're going to keep injecting heroin, this is what's going to happen to you" ends up with poor outcomes. Very poor. Why? They are not in a place to hear that. Genuineness and honesty are an important part of relational paradigms. However, if you don't have the trust of a user, it won't be received.

In my life, I've had a handful of occasions where someone has been very direct with me, enough to change the trajectory of my life. It's important to know who those three people were: an uncle, a parent, and a coach. In all three instances, I knew that they were out for my best welfare, and would still love or care for me, even if I said, "No." Blunt advice and direct confrontation has its place. But you have to have the relationship to make these direct advances successful.

I wonder sometimes if that isn't why harm reduction hasn't gained more traction in the industry. It's easy to say, "I can't work with you if you're not going to be sober." Because, to stay open and have hope, means there's more anxiety, more uncertainty. If a person is in bad shape, it's probably going to be really hard to make them better. But to give in and say there's "no hope" takes all the anxiety away from the helper, because the horizon is known. With pessimism, there's no anxiousness, because you already have fixed the outcome (failure). But if [you] take a hopeful stance, regardless of the current situation to think *some* progress could be made—now you must occupy a place of uncertainty, all of which are harder on the helper—it creates trepidation.

One of the important issues (according to Miller & Rollnick) about being able to use motivational interviewing correctly is divorcing yourself from the consequences of a personal situation. As a treatment provider, I need to be able to relinquish control. I have to be able to turn it over to that person. Why would I dominate and set up a plan that I create? I'm not the one who's going to be doing the changing. Yikes. I'm the central actor in this?

Harm reduction needs to be an accepted pathway for improved health; it needs a seat at the table, across all disciplines. Legal health, psychological health, physical health. If you want to run an abstinence-only drug court, fine. But if you find someone who is going to continue using and wants to reduce their risks, then we bring them over to someone who is adept at doing that type of work.

We can't use sobriety as a benchmark for whether someone is worthy of being treated with kindness. Can we say, "Well, since you refuse to be abstinent, we're not going to help you" and have no options or alternatives for them? No recommendations of where they *might go*?

I want people to understand how much of a brain disease addiction truly is. To treat that, we need a fuller understanding of human motivation and the process of behavioral change. I also wish more people in the industry understood treatment cannot be imposed on another. We must offer the full spectrum of services to people coming in our door. And sometimes we, as therapeutic providers, can do more harm if we're not willing to do that. To say, "Well, at least I tried—I guess they weren't ready" doesn't cut it. Not if we made things worse for that individual because of what we did. Psychotherapeutic? How about Psychonoxious. Don't violate the maxim "First, Do No Harm."

At the end of the day, any provider must be able to look at themselves in the mirror and say, "I did all I could." That means using *all seats* at the table, via more options, differing referrals, increasing our alternatives. This epidemic calls us to move out of our boxes.

Michael can be reached at mike.clark.mi@gmail.com

SUSAN COLLINS

When I went to college, I knew exactly what I wanted to do: become a clinical psychologist. I am now a licensed clinical psychologist in Washington State. I was trained to do assessments that all clinical psychologists do for depression and anxiety disorders, as well as provide treatment for those disorders, but my primary focus over the past twenty-five years is working with assessing, treating, and researching addictive behaviors. The study of addictive behaviors is also very personal as it is for so many of us in this field.

I grew up in a family with the intergenerational experience of substance use disorder and addictive behaviors. Both my mother and my father and their families struggled with addictive behaviors, and I married into such a family as well. When I was fourteen or fifteen years old (and training to become a professional ballet dancer), I developed an eating disorder. Around the time I developed that eating disorder, I also had my first drink and soon after started using other drugs as well. I entered treatment for my eating disorder and afterwards ended up in a 12 Step group for eating disorders, Overeaters Anonymous, where I got my first sponsor. It was while attending that first 12 Step group (when I was about sixteen) that I realized pretty quickly that while I was going to meetings for eating disorders, I had all these other addictions going on at the same time; I was really struggling. I remember being obsessed every day with all sorts of psychic pain, asking myself how I could I make it go away.

I danced until I was seventeen when I had a car accident, and that event made me question what I was doing about a lot of things. Ultimately, I decided not to become a ballet dancer. I said to myself, "I guess I'm going to college." I decided that if I was going to go to college, the only career path I was interested in choosing was to figure out why my family and I were so messed up, like many who wind up working in the field of addiction.

I applied for graduate school knowing exactly what I was going to do: be an addiction counselor so I could help other people with problems like mine. I still hadn't fully resolved my issues, but I really felt like that was the right pathway. However, I was counseled by my mentor not to talk about my own struggles with addictive behaviors, not even to mention my family's struggles, because it would be, and I quote, "a red flag." I love my mentors and sadly they were right at the time. If you were an academic, if you were a clinician, you could not have your own struggles. That wasn't okay. As academics and clinicians, we were expected to be healthy and whole and perfect, because we were going to help others; *they* were the who were "sick and problematic," right? What a way to start a career!

Over the next decade, my eating disorder did resolve, and I would credit 12 Step for some of that. I also credit good psychotherapy and the eating disorders treatments I went through. But there was first an epiphany that many of us with addictive behaviors are familiar with. While bending over a toilet and vomiting on one particular but not very notable day, I remember saying to myself, "What am I doing? This has got to stop." It didn't all suddenly resolve that day, but I finally felt like I needed to stop. It took me some years after that to develop a really healthy relationship with food, but I was able to do it eventually. Then I could start looking at my other addictive behaviors.

I grew up in the field, as we all did in a certain time, as an abstinence-only substance use treatment counselor. As part of my training, I learned 12 Step Facilitation, CBT, and I used Motivational Interviewing, all to help aid people's transitions from intensive outpatient (IOP) to outpatient treatment and to aftercare. The focus was on relapse prevention. We were supposed to help people get sober and stay sober.

In school, I had learned all these fancy therapeutic techniques to provide treatment for the people that came in. The first thing I was asked to do when I went on an internship was to put on rubber gloves and stand in the bathroom and watch women pee. That baffled me. I also wondered *why* we were doing it. I was told that when the results came back from those urine toxicology tests, I was to write a letter to the judge or the Department of Children and Families or the probation officer and give them the results. I did what I was asked even though I didn't like doing it. It wasn't until years later that I read about mass incarceration, and I realized that I contributed to that. That was me: I wrote those letters. I became a de facto arm of the criminal justice system. When did I train for that? When was I given informed consent around that? I was shocked and disgusted.

I first really began to think more seriously about the kind of treatment people receive in rehabs while I was working with folks experiencing homelessness and severe substance use disorders. We learned through that research that the people we were working with had gone through abstinence-based treatment a mean of sixteen times. I remember talking to these participants about their treatment experiences, and that's when I really started to understand the anger they were feeling about treatment and towards us, treatment providers. It made me think, "What are we doing?" Clearly, we weren't helping the most severely impacted people in the ways that we intended. And relapse prevention wasn't really catching fire with these folks. I started thinking maybe we should be asking them, the clients, what they want out of treatment, [questioning] how we failed them as treatment providers. Maybe we should be saying, "You're not 'treatment failures'; maybe the system has just failed you."

It was those conversations over a period of years that started to get me really curious about what we could do differently. We started to ask people, "What would you want to see happen for yourself, if you could design treatment in your own vision? What would that look like?" And that led Seema Clifasefi, a colleague of mine, and I to write a series of NIH grants where we then co-created that kind of treatment—harm reduction treatment—with people with lived or living experience in substance use. And we tested that through randomized clinical controlled trials that saw positive effects in terms of engagement as well as a reduction in substance-related harm, even a reduction in use. Paradoxically, we weren't asking people to change their drug use patterns, we were just asking them what they wanted to happen for themselves regarding their lives, including their substance use. After the fifteen plus years that Seema and I have been doing this work, the real gift is being able to carry forward what these clients and community members and patients gave me—gave us—and that's what they said in our research studies: "Yeah I'm doing this for the twenty bucks that you give me, but I'm also doing this because I really want other people to not have to go through what I've gone through, or have better care than I had." I want to be sure we pay that forward and we make a change for the better.

Our job became to teach participants ways they could stay safer and healthier and celebrate their own ways of staying safer and healthier. We found that people who started treatment on their own terms and on their own timeline could reduce their use. Ironically, it was this work that finally led me to finish working on addictive behaviors of my own that were still around.

My family history was heavy on alcohol. It was all a big part of our culture. That's just what people did. But my family seemed to struggle more to manage the consequences. My grandfather, a WW2 veteran, was very much involved in that first generation of AA. He involved his whole life in AA, but still vacillated between periods of sobriety and periods of extremely heavy drinking. This struggle shaped my family of origin and many of us have gone on to struggle with our substance use and other addictive behaviors. As mentioned, I then married into such a family that had its own separate set of issues with alcohol and other drug use. Even as my eating disorders and drug use had resolved at that point, my drinking had continued. I used harm reduction for many, many years, and was very high functioning with my alcohol use. Then, I had my daughter. After mostly abstaining from drinking while I was pregnant, I found myself slowly drinking more heavily than I had been. I had long been a daily drinker, but now I would drink long into the night, after everyone had gone to sleep.

Over time, I started to realize that I could not be the mother that I wanted to be drinking like I was. I also experienced the recurrence of alcohol-induced gastritis that was very painful and made it hard to eat. One day, I wound up in urgent care, and the doctor came in and laced his fingers together and said, "I think you know what I'm going to say, Miss Collins: You're an alcoholic, and you've got to quit drinking if you want things to get better." And naturally because of my knowledge of addiction, I said to him, "I'm not an alcoholic. That diagnosis hasn't existed since the DSM II. So, you're off base." Well, that conversation sure didn't go as he expected. But I had already been pretty clear that I needed to make a change in my relationship to alcohol.

I think it was the frustration after that experience in healthcare about my alcohol use, as well as hearing this from many others over my decades in the field that have made me clear that abstinence-only treatment cannot be the only thing we have on offer. Of course, I still think there's a place for 12 Step facilitation and CBT and more because, if I'm truly going to meet all patients where they're at, we need to offer lots of options

To me harm reduction is a large set of compassionate and pragmatic approaches that aim to help people reduce their substance related harm and improve their quality of life without requiring abstinence or even use reduction. It helped me when I first started learning about harm reduction from my late mentor, Alan Marlatt, to go through his work and his writings, and of course his counsel at the time. He helped me understand we can approach harm reduction from very different places in the system. Some people are going to work on harm-reduction policy, some people are going to work on population-based messaging around reduction. Some people are going to work with community-level interventions, like Housing First, or managed alcohol programs, or syringe service programs. And some people are going to work on the individual level, like me as a psychotherapist. Sometimes, as harm reductionists, we can work across all those domains. We might influence policy with our research with individual treatments. Being open to doing more than just what our job description is, that's also part of harm reduction.

What I've struggled with the most in this work is when it feels like some parts of society wants to pit harm reduction against abstinence, and it becomes really politicized in a way that's counterproductive for everybody involved. I'm reminded of an interview I was asked to do with a conservative talk radio show, maybe a year and a half ago or so. It was going to be presented as me—the wild, liberal, left, progressive, harm reductionist—versus a person with lived experience who is a peer now and abstinence based. The usual myths were thrown out like "harm reduction kills," very extreme, and the show people tried to put it in that way. We were also both women, and the show producers were all men so there was also a bit of sexism involved. It felt like "let's have a cat fight between the right and the left on this!" The other woman and I were very disappointed by all this and when she and I ended up agreeing a lot, the host seemed disappointed. That's not what they wanted. Sometimes I think that's what we are asked to do, have some kind of fireworks, like it's abstinence against harm reduction, and I don't think it is. I really feel we should be meeting people where they're at, providing people and families with a menu of options so that they can start their recovery journey wherever they are; they are not required to be a certain way or to meet a certain milestone before they can get help. Right now, I'm returning home from an Overdose Awareness Day event in Seattle where one family member who started a nonprofit shared about the loss of their son to overdose. They said no one ever talked to them about harm reduction as an option to possibly help their son, and she felt that conversation could have saved his life. That's what frustrates me about our system: We don't present all the options. This mom said her son was required to do sober living, and he overdosed there. Where was the harm reduction here? I really think harm reduction says you can be sober. That's one path, but it's not the only path. We shouldn't save recovery only for people who are ready to get sober. We need to have recovery options available for people wherever they are—and for families wherever they are too.

Harm reduction needs to be offered in all phases of treatment if we're really going to save lives. I have these amazing colleagues Caleb Banta Green and Mandy Owens at the University of Washington, and they're working with the Washington State legislature right now to require treatment programs to tell people about *all* of the evidence-based options that are available—harm reduction, including medications—and not just require sobriety and no other options for people. I mean many treatment agencies aren't even telling people that there are medications that could help them avoid cravings and urges, help them stabilize wherever they are on a substance use continuum. What I want to see now is that those same treatment agencies have to talk about harm reduction as an evidence-based treatment option. I want us to have harm reduction fully integrated into our treatment system that all substance use disorders providers—addiction psychologists, addiction medicine doctors, addiction psychiatrists, anyone serving these folks—all need to be trained in harm reduction, alongside 12 Step facilitation, alongside CBT, alongside MI and more. We really need to know about substances, how to talk to people about safer use strategies, how to talk about harm reduction goal setting really explicitly. And we need to be able to talk to families about that too. This is so personal for me, as well as professional. You know, if I could be a part of that dream coming true, of integrating harm reduction into our healthcare systems, I'd feel like I've made my grandfather proud. I'd happily retire on that happening. If we can do that, then my work here is done.

Susan be reached at https://depts.washington.edu/harrtlab

JENNIFER FERNANDEZ

I always say that harm reduction chose me! I was a pre-doctoral psychology intern looking for a practicum placement and the Harm Reduction Therapy Center (HRTC) was one of the options. I thought, "Sure, why not? Addiction seems interesting enough." Clearly, I didn't know a thing about addictions and how incredibly complex they are to treat. I didn't have any formal training in addiction at that point either, just one five-hour course as part of my doctoral program. I have a personal history of addiction in my family, but it wasn't immediately clear to me that this was something I needed to address within myself as I began helping others navigate their own struggles. Perri [Franskoviak] conducted my interview and explained what they did at the HRTC, how they approached addiction, and it all made perfect sense to me!

Harm reduction psychotherapy resonated with me because it mirrored how I observed drug use around me—acknowledging both its benefits and risks. My personal experiences with drug use, particularly the positive outcomes I found through psychedelic exploration, made HRT a natural fit with my existing view of substance use and my commitment to a human-centered approach. Also, the concept of "radical compassion" in HRT resonated with my desire to work relationally with everyone I encountered, and continue to see, as a clinical psychologist. The final point Perri shared during our interview about HRT that hit hard was my long standing fascination with neuroscience, seeing the brain as a kind of "last frontier." There's so much about the brain that we have yet to discover and that has always been very intriguing to me. I appreciate how effective addiction treatment seamlessly combines neuroscience with the relational dynamics of the therapeutic process. HRT was the perfect fit for my curious mind and I've never looked back. I've been a committed harm reductionist since that interview in 2009. This experience also led me to do my dissertation on harm reduction psychotherapy, and I have dedicated myself to the practice of HRT since.

Today, when I think about harm reduction, I conceptualize it as three things:

1) respect for others, 2) humility in the face of intense challenge and distress, and 3) a celebration of the change process. I believe these factors are crucial in the work I do with clients, as they also help shift their self-perception as someone struggling with addiction—someone wanting to make a different choice and unable to do so. It is truly transformative when I'm able to bring that respect and humility to the complexity of addiction and to really celebrate *any* positive change, anything at all, no matter how incremental it is. I have the privilege of being a strong advocate and cheerleader for those transformative moments that make a significant difference in people's journeys through the challenge of addiction. I also see how this

way of being with people gives them hope after they come to us feeling incredibly hopeless, broken, stigmatized, and ashamed.

I bring this same spirit to my work with clients who aren't seeking help for substance misuse but may be dealing with process addictions or other things like major depressive disorder, for example. Whatever they bring, I show up with that same respect, humility, and celebration of the change process—which by the way is an incredibly difficult process. The therapeutic work we do can be truly transformative for everyone.

Any change process is rarely quick. It's almost always messy and difficult, presenting challenges for us as therapists *and* the individuals we're supporting. That's where the part about humility has been really important to my work in HRT. When I was a younger therapist, I used to think, "I can change this person," much like we sometimes believe in our personal relationships. But over time, I learned that there are forces and processes far bigger than us, which we need to respect, understand, and approach with curiosity. I think bringing curiosity to any relationship helps. And in HRT it can also help reduce the "change" or intensity associated with change, making the process smoother.

Most people don't understand what harm reduction is, and certainly not HRT. Many people have a misconception of it. They accuse us of enabling, colluding with people who use drugs, or simply standing by as people harm themselves. I really wish others could see it as a practice of *radical compassion*. Radical compassion is the mindset or relational atmosphere we cultivate to effectively engage with folks, particularly those who use substances. When I'm training and consulting with other therapists, I try to impart this way of working with clients as well as the kind of environment we need to create in which change can happen. Here in the United States and in Western culture, I think of Jesus as the most popular figurehead of compassion, the way he unconditionally loved all people. He accepted everyone *radically.* And so this ethos of "wherever you're at, whoever you are, I'm just going to meet you there" is at the core of harm reduction and harm reduction psychotherapy. And of all effective psychotherapy, frankly.

Now, there are times when I *can't* meet people where they're at and I have an ethical obligation to be aware of those times. I have to be able to acknowledge that it's not a good fit or that this isn't the right patient population or setting for me. And most importantly, *that's on me;* that's *my* stuff getting in the way of the work, not theirs. Just having that self-awareness about where you are able to give that compassion unconditionally, and where you aren't, is essential as a provider, regardless of the context you're working in.

I wish people could see harm reduction more as a spiritual practice, or at least in that vein. In HRT, I have to consciously and intentionally work to keep my heart open, actively recognizing and setting aside my biases and judgments as much as possible to be able to give the person I'm working with an experience of true *unconditional love, unconditional positive regard.* This work really is unconditional love. And that spirit feeds *me* just as much as it helps the other person.

I would also like to see more of this spirit, harm reduction as unconditional love, in how we work with people in all addiction treatment. For me, this unconditional love would include more involvement of the family or the chosen family, because one's biological family is not always safe to include in treatment. In all mental health treatment, it's essential to approach the whole person within the context of their existing systems. However, with addiction, there are additional layers to consider—particularly the pervasive elements of shame, isolation, and disconnection. So involving a person's family of origin, chosen family, community, or other significant individuals in their life is crucial to their process of change and to gaining a deeper understanding of their behavior. That's also part of harm reduction and HRT.

Lastly, I believe harm reduction and HRT should prioritize family involvement, integrating them throughout the addiction treatment process. This includes their participation in assessments, ongoing support, and providing accurate psychoeducation about addiction and the family's role in recovery. Additionally, families should be educated about the change process as part of aftercare—basically from "soup to nuts!" It would be wonderful to have this integrated into HRT, but it's pretty rare. I think it's more acceptable to involve families with teens and I see a lot more integration between teens and their parents. I don't know why we think adults don't need that same level of relational support. I'd love to see someone develop a harm reduction family therapy! Harm reduction psychotherapy encourages you to consider the broader systems and environments that shape the life of the person you're working with. We need an addiction treatment that's focused on the family and bridges some of the existing modalities to help understand the etiology and maintenance of whatever the addictive disorder may be, and to bring in the family as part of those interventions or strategies. We've got to let the family into this journey we call *treatment and recovery* if we're to see change that lasts. Perhaps this is the last piece of HRT that's been missing to some degree. Perhaps it's our role to guide families in becoming that source of unconditional love they deeply wish to provide for their loved ones and themselves, fostering true healing from the effects of addiction. And I think Harm Reduction Psychotherapy is the perfect vehicle for this change.

Jennifer can be reached at jennifer@cacenterforchange.com
https://cacenterforchange.com

PERRI FRANSKOVIAK

'm thinking about how I came to harm reduction and realizing that it's really hard for me to put a start point on it. I guess I came to harm reduction when I was in graduate school, getting my Masters degree in Denver and I was in a practicum at the Malcolm X Mental Health Center. I had seen this client for an intake who was presenting with intense symptoms of depression: poor sleep, difficulty concentrating, and self-esteem that was in the basement. He's what we would now call "working poor." He'd lost his job—maybe he'd gotten laid off—and he just couldn't find a foothold for himself. He started drinking. I think his drinking had been a problem in the past, but he had been able to get a handle on it and drink more moderately, so it wasn't impacting his life until he began running into lot of trouble getting hired again. We talked a little bit about his relationship to alcohol and how he knew he had to slow down, and that it was the only thing that was keeping him going for now. This was in the late '80s, and there was still so little known about co-occurring disorders. But I do remember being really curious: I knew alcohol was a depressant and he was clearly clinically depressed and thinking, "so how do drinking and depression work together?"

So fast forward, I presented this client to my supervisor who was the co-director of the mental health center. I was looking forward to getting to work with him, one of my first clients, and to my surprise she said to me, "Oh, no, he has to wait a year before he can come in for therapy because he's drinking." Wait, that made no sense to me. I mean, how could this man work on his relationship to alcohol without getting treatment for his depression? And vice versa? Anyway, that just made no sense to me at all. After my practicum, I got hired by the same mental health center and that client returned a year later, and you know what? He stopped drinking! Wow. And he wanted to come back and see me! Wow. So that was one beginning point for me come to harm reduction.

Another point at which I came to harm reduction was when I was working at another community mental health center in Denver. I was working on the emergency psychiatric team where we saw people coming in from the community who needed emergency psychiatric services. Sometimes the police would bring in non-violent folks for us to assess. We'd also get called to local hospitals to go out and assess people who did not already have a therapist in the community or at a mental health center in the Denver area. One of the things we would do on the emergency team was making connections with other treatment providers who would work with our clients. We were also connected to the Community Support Program, which was for folks with severe mental illness. These clients had diagnoses like schizophrenia, bipolar disorder, major depression with psychotic features. There was a program in Denver called Arapahoe House—a program for folks living with both the mental illness of drug use and other mental illnesses like depression, PTSD, crippling anxiety, and psychosis. They wanted someone from our team to come in once a month and sit with them in their team meeting just so there could be a liaison between our two agencies. Our supervisor asked for a volunteer to go to Arapahoe House for these monthly meetings and nobody volunteered. No one was interested. So, I volunteered. This experience was really the beginning for me of starting to get a sense of how there's no such thing as just a substance use disorder or just a mental health disorder. They're all in the same book. And not only that, but they're all on the same page, and in the same person.

I have lived through the era where these were separate systems, and now they're coming together more, but there's still a disjunction between the two worlds: substance use disorder on the one hand and mental health on the other. Unfortunately many providers still want to cut people into quarters, or halves, and not treat the whole person.

That was really my start in harm reduction therapy. Also, I have a very personal experience with alcohol and other drug use in that my parents were killed by a drunk driver, a man who had several previous drunk driving offenses. And you know, it wasn't until I was pretty far down the road into my career—by the time I'd been out here in California at least ten years—that I began to see the direction I was heading in, working with drug users. You don't really perceive that you're on a path, you just kind of take the next opportunity that comes up, and the next and the next. But I began to realize that these really are my people. I saw something of myself in those folks who, as Patt Denning would say, "... were willing to be worried about their drug and alcohol use." And I started thinking, "Isn't this interesting? People are opening up to me, and something's transforming in me as well.

Wow." At the time I had the lofty aspirations of someone young in her career of wanting to make the world a better place for everyone, one person at a time. Now I see that we're all suffering in one way or another, running game and having it run on us, and that we need attunement to take the first steps toward making a change.

All this leads me to think about how I define harm reduction today. The first thing that comes to mind about harm reduction is that it's a process. *Harm reduction is a process.* I mean, you can talk about it in terms of outcomes: we want to reduce harm. Countless studies have been done measuring drug and alcohol use during and after treatment, as well as expanding the measurements beyond just alcohol and other drug use such as looking at quality of life, housing, physical health, and mental health. Harm reduction applies to everything. It's about all kinds of behaviors. Harm reduction is a process of being open to how each one of us defines harm and how we define success.

I would also have to say that one of my deepest identities is in being a therapist, a helper, so to me, harm reduction is a process of the helper being open to difference. By that, I mean really opening up and getting curious and bringing in warmth toward another person's experience, which is always going to be different from ours. But particularly being as open as we possibly can be. Also, harm reduction is about us getting consultation, supervision, all the things that help us keep our boundaries more *open* to other people who will always activate us. And we do get activated. I mean, we're all human beings, we have a nervous system. That means if I am being open and track when I'm not, so many amazing things can happen. And the client gets to be where they are. They don't have to be where we want or need them to be. They get to be just where they are. They get to get be seen as someone with agency and dignity. We get to be humble. I'm continually being humbled in my work as a therapist. I think I know something and then the next words out of my client's mouth will take me in a completely different direction. People get to feel valued in harm reduction work. I strongly believe that no change takes place outside of a relationship, even if it's just a relationship in our mind—an internalized object relationship. The longer I do this work, the more apparent it becomes to me that the line between client and clinician is in many ways just gossamer thin.

It's been great to see harm reduction being discussed more and strategies being used now. I'd also like to see better training in general but especially in harm reduction therapy. I think our academic programs are still training people that substance use is over here, and mental health is over there. I mean, my god, we know that substance use is a mental health disorder. It's all in the DSM! So I think we need more and better training in the academic world. And I think in terms of treatment, we need to get the 12 Steps the FUCK OUT of treatment programs. 12 Step is not treatment and was never intended to be. AA itself says that it's a program of support not treatment and yet, that's what we've done. And what we still do. I think we do that to make things simpler for ourselves as practitioners and to push away the things— the people—that activate us and make us feel un-comfortable. So back to that inner transformation. We have to be open to being changed by the folks we work with.

I would like to see treatment programs that are actually built on evidence-based practices. I think we really need to make a de-marcation between support and treatment. I'd like to see more therapy in treatment, not just skill building groups and didactic or psychosocial groups. We need more therapy, where people get to sit with another person. Where they get to develop a trusting relationship so that they can share some of the deep-down stuff that maybe makes it difficult for them to make changes in their life, and to have all of that be normalized.

We have such an unwieldy healthcare system. Unfortunately, we have privatized it and made it a money-making venture. Healthcare is a for profit industry in the US. I think that's a mistake. I think if you're truly interested in investing in your country, you need to invest in the health of your people. I mean, we are the greatest resource in this country, just as the population of any country is. This may be pie in the sky but I'd really like to see a model, like the National Health Service in the UK here in the US. We've already got that in Medicare. You can call it socialized medicine. I know that word is a hot potato with certain subgroups in our country at this time, but that's the model I'd like to see. But failing that, I'd like the insurance companies to really cover more in terms of mental health treatment and provide much more generous benefits for getting mental health treatment for alcohol and other drug use, and for any self-harming behavior treated. People cry out for mental health treatment after a mass shooting, but we still don't prioritize it. The latest shooting fades away, and we don't follow through. It's so deep. It's one of those systemic issues like white supremacy and class supremacy that we haven't yet figured out how to change. We need our scapegoats apparently.

So those are big global changes I'd love to see. I'd really like to see everybody who is working in any kind of a therapeutic role be trained in harm reduction. It's really based on Carl Rogers' work. It should be taught like a very basic kind of client-centered model. It should be taught as naturally as we teach those good rapport building skills in graduate programs. We also need more training on how to manage our own feelings as they come up, and what kind of information is contained in them. What can we learn about ourselves and about the person or persons we're working with?

Lastly, I think what I'd like people to know about harm reduction work is that it's nothing special. To me, it's really about just being a good human being, a good citizen, a good community member. It involves being willing to open our boundaries to something that's different from ourselves. Bring in some curiosity and be willing to be changed in the process. Each human encounter changes the people that are involved. It's an infinite number of interactions that are taking place right in this moment, and they're changing every human being connected to them. And at its core, that's what harm reduction is.

Perri can be reached at pfranskoviak@gmail.com

ROBB FULGHAM

I have many titles, but the one I normally go by is "Supervising Substance Use Disorder Counselor," although I supervise all of the programs plus adult case management. My journey has been an interesting ride. I was twenty-six when I went into a county program. At the time, everything was about 12 Steps meetings. There were no other options. I had a sponsor who'd pick me up to take me to a meeting, and then we're out there selling our product like it was Amway. You have newcomers entering, and the seasoned pro. It was very much like a pyramid scheme. I just remember thinking, "This is weird."

I started to question the labeling, because it felt stigmatizing. My opposition to the traditional recovery approach didn't make me very popular. I didn't make big waves. I was probably ten years clean when I left that all behind. Personally, I didn't feel like an addict anymore. I'd abstained for over a decade. I felt like a different person. Using never crossed my mind. I didn't drink, I didn't use, so why would I keep attending AA? As you know, AA/NA will answer: once an addict, always an addict. It's a lifelong process. And, sorry, but I believe in recovery—that people can get better if they really want to.

So, no, I did not identify with that 12 Step approach.

It wasn't until around the early 2000s that you started to hear the term "harm reduction." I was working in the industry at this time, helping others get their lives back on track. I was bringing literature to work, different books that espoused new approaches to treatment. The cool part was? I didn't get a lot of pushback. I was fortunate to work with others who could keep an open mind, say, "Hey, if this or that works, and it's *not* part of the 12 Step model, who cares? It works!"

Overall, it hasn't been a difficult transition. These days, people meet the client with a new attitude: do no harm. Let's keep people safe. They realize that *all* recovery doesn't neatly fit in a box. Recovery comprises a spectrum of ideas and philosophies. Thankfully, with harm reduction, we are *finally* moving away from an "one size fits all" approach.

That's not to say I didn't experience *any* pushback. It's human nature to be apprehensive of change. This goes for addicts *and* some counselors too. Change is scary! Luckily, I had people around me who had been sober for a while, backing me up.

One of the first things I did when they put me in charge in 2013, I said, "Wait a minute! The courts can't mandate meetings anymore because it's church. Freedom of religion. So we're not going to either!" We sat around the table, and we expanded the idea, and we changed it to community support. We had people volunteering for Habitat for Humanity. Because we were all using this open-minded angle, it helped gel our mission statement, at the center of which was, and remains: do the client no harm.

Of course 12 Step is still very prevalent. It's only been over the last eight to ten years that we got Celebrate Recovery. The mental health department, a number of years ago, started a SAMI (substance abuse, mental illness) group. The program was really popular for a while, but it died out. 12 Step programs, to their credit, have proven to have staying power. Because they *do* work for many. I'm interested in the ones whom it doesn't help. For me, that brings recovery back to harm reduction.

About ten years ago, I was standing on the outside of our building. I'm looking up at the big sign that said, "Substance Abuse Programs." And I grabbed a screwdriver and I took it off. It's still sitting behind my desk. Now, it just says "Behavioral Health." It's a new—and in my opinion— better way to view the changes one has to make if he/she/they want to recover. Sometimes it's all about opening up your eyes and viewing the world differently.

We recently applied for a grant. In the next few years, we'll get a single building, which will help consolidate efforts. Right now all our work is spread across several buildings.

One of my first duties was getting a report on diagnosis from the Mental Health Department. And there were probably almost three hundred substance-use disorder diagnoses of clients that had not even been referred. I had a meeting with all the clinicians. I said I need an explanation. I'm not questioning your authority or professionalism in the field, but why would you do this (label them as having a disorder) and not refer them for services? And it all just came down to money. We were cash pay; they were MediCal. They straight up said, "We don't want to deal with that." Now, we take MediCal and it's changing, we regularly now get referrals.

We're across the street from the local hospital. Luckily, my wife is the social worker there. And by default, because they never hired a substance use navigator, she's it.

How it works is, I get a I get a fax or an encrypted email, with a signed release, saying this person wants to talk to somebody. Either I, or one of my staff, we go over to the hospital. And yeah, it's non-billable. But you know what? I want to keep people alive more than I care about making money.

So much of healthcare, including substance-use treatments, gets caught up in the bureaucracy of the politics of wellness. We could get the hospital certified. It would be funded right now. But then many of these people wouldn't get seen, couldn't get help. How can you help someone if you never contact them?

We're the only country that calls it "abuse" anyway. Everybody else calls it "misuse." This is a casualty of the War on Drugs, and I think that really ties into self-image, the stigma, how a drug user is treated and views him or herself. Because once I had dealt with my traumas, and my situations, and you know, family stuff, I had no desire to use. It just went away. Which 12 Step and AA/NA will tell you isn't possible. But it is! Who wants to be "sick" forever? It makes you feel hopeless, and it affects a person's self-esteem.

One of my best friends in the whole world just retired. He'd always say, "I'm just an old dope fiend." And that's valid too. That's how he absolutely feels. But how sad is that? I remember a conversation we had a few years ago, and I said, "I see myself as normal. Using doesn't even come into play for me." And he was shocked. He said, "When I tell somebody that I get, well, then you weren't a real addict." Can you imagine? I told him, "We're talking about having ten, twenty, thirty years clean." Why still view yourself in such a negative light with expressions like "I'm just an old dope fiend?"

Yes, I personally believe treatment is a lifelong process, in the sense that the proclivity to use *is* in you. But also if you heal the trauma, it no longer harms you, or its impact is lessened and you can deal with life without resorting to constantly needing to numb emotions. You change, you become someone else, and you move on with your life. Maybe those lessons that you learned when you were out there can be put into practice or used for good? I don't think anyone needs to sit in a room thirty years after the fact and rehash decades-old baggage.

I want to keep people safe and alive. And if they need somebody to hold their hand, great! You hold their hand. And if someone else feels like they want to go to a Big Book study, fantastic. You do you! But recovery also means keeping an open mind. I couldn't ever go, "Oh, well, it's needle exchange! That's encouraging people to use!" No, those are programs based on harm reduction, keeping people alive. I think for me, that's just the core of it.

Right now, the big scare is fentanyl. So, we have strips to test for it. We carry a supply of Narcan, too, as well as local MD's who prescribe buprenorphine. Whatever you need to get better and stay safe—*that's* what we're here for.

I can tell you this, the demographics of Calaveras County are predominantly conservative, retired folks. We do face opposition. That being said, we just got additional funding. We already have the crisis mobile unit for behavioral health. That's part of it. Education is a huge part of it.

It wasn't long ago that the suggestion to put someone on methadone was seen as a resignation of failure almost. Many in the recovery community were, like, "Oh, no I don't believe in that." But in my little neck of the woods, that's everybody's go-to. If that's the best route for a patient, we ask, "How do we get them medication?"

The path to recovery is an individual journey. For some that means AA and 12 Step, others harm reduction, another abstinence. Different strokes, different folks. What do *you* need? What do *you* need *today*? And how can I help you get it? Let's move forward, you know, because it's gonna look completely different for virtually everybody.

Robb can be reached at fulgham@gmail.com

REID HESTER

I got interested in psychology when I was a junior at the University of Washington in Seattle. Prior to that I was an English major. I really had to put a lot of effort into finishing up my psychology major in the latter half of my four years. When I completed that, I was burned out. I did my senior thesis and the paper was published in a peer reviewed journal. Afterwards, I needed to take a break and I took a year off and spent four months backpacking through Europe. When I got back, I went to the Psychology Department at UW to see what research projects were going on. That's what I ran into Alan Marlatt. Alan had just come down from the University of British Columbia in Vancouver.

I volunteered to be a confederate[1] in one of his first drinking studies that looked at the effects of modeling on people's drinking. And that was a Caudill & Marlatt paper that came out sometime around 1974. In the study I posed as a regular college student. For the study, ostensibly a taste-test task, you

1. In a research experiment confederates are individuals who seem to be participants but in reality are part of the research team. They essentially trick real participants into thinking they are fellow participants.

273

were allowed to drink as much as you wanted over the course of fifteen minutes. In the high consumption (vs. low), I would drink twenty-five ounces in fifteen minutes. In light of this they diluted my red wine with grape juice. What researchers discovered was if I drank a lot, the other participant drank a lot; if I drank a little, the other student followed suit.

That was the modeling behavior hypothesis. This launched a series of studies by Barry Caudill and others—looking at what sort of influence social interactions and social context has on drinking.

Alan Marlatt actually had a drinking lab in his psychology department's basement for various experiments. When I was getting ready to go to Washington State University for graduate school, he told me to look up Warren Garlington, who was a psychology professor there. Warren was working on concepts centered around controlled drinking. When I met Warren, we got along splendidly. I became a predoc fellow in his alcohol training program, which focused on moderate drinking protocols. This triggered a whole sequence of events. As I was preparing for my internship in Albuquerque, New Mexico, Warren suggested I connect with Bill Miller, who was in the psychology department at the University of New Mexico.

Bill and I decided to work together. At that point, there had been quite a bit of literature on alcohol treatment that had taken place in the previous ten years—basically the entire seventies decade. Bill and I began to review much of this literature, searching for the most effective strategies regarding alcoholism and treatment. One of the top ones was brief interventions. Also, moderate moderation training and community reinforcement approaches were proven to work. Those three were consistent strains, along with social skills training.

Bill eventually went on sabbaticals, which took him to first to Norway then to Sydney, Australia. And that's where he ran into Steve Rollnick. Steve had read Bill's research and findings. Steve suggested they collaborate on a book. Bill, in his usual collaborative fashion, jumped at the opportunity. This is how the first edition of *Motivational Interviewing* was born. I'm proud to say that I was the one who suggested that he go to Australia or New Zealand for a sabbatical.

While Bill was in Australia, I took over supervising his grad students. This was before email became a thing. He and I continued to collaborate, but the process was different back then. We worked around the time zones and miles between us, and were able to put together workshops and trainings, as well as additional research studies together. We had a wonderful collegial relationship for many years. I was fortunate to work with and learn from pioneers like Alan Marlatt, Warren Garlington, and Bill Miller.

In the late seventies, Bill put on an international conference up in Taos, New Mexico—the first such conference on the treatment of addictive behaviors. I got to meet many of the founding members of clinical research community.

In the mid-eighties, a project officer at the National Institute on Alcohol Abuse and Alcoholism (NIAAA) approached me following a talk I gave on treatment effectiveness. He told me about NIAAA's new funding mechanism centered around small business and innovative research. He wanted me to submit a proposal. I put together a proposal, and they funded it to develop my first software program, which was a behavioral self-control program for Windows.

Prior to this I had been treating DWI offenders using an eight week group training protocol that Bill Miller had developed. As the questions these clients often asked came up over and over again, I began thinking about how this was something that a computer could do. Regular computer use was still in its infancy. But the idea was an early variation on what Google and other search engines would become. You ask the questions, you receive a response. The first software program was straight forward, a moderate drinking protocol. That evolved over time.

Bill and I were known to the parole officers. We were acquainted with the judges who would hand down sentencing. We had evidence that first-time offenders were typically not seriously dependent and the judges were open to our proposal to teach them harm reduction skills. That was how I got involved with the DWI population.

After developing the Drinker's Checkup in the late nineties, we implemented it in the DWI program up in Farmington, New Mexico, a thirty-day, inpatient, residential treatment program. It's basically in a jail. A very nice jail. But still a jail. They started using our drinkers checkup as a CD ROM-based Windows program.

We found reductions in drinking, and continued our research through the nineties and into the early 2000s. By now computer use was more prevalent, and we moved our program into a web application. We had a contract with the state (New Mexico) to do trainings and provide the software applications to them. In doing so, we assumed that along with workshops, we could send therapists off and they'd be successful on their own. Unfortunately, that was not the case. We realized we needed a more hands-on approach.

And the challenge was (and is still) that there are so many different ways that it can go sideways. With implementation, you must have the stakeholders on board, the people who make the decisions to continue the program or not continue the program after the funding is approved. You have to train the personnel and get them on board. And then you have to continue to provide support and supervision. And even if you do have people who are on board with your ideas, the funding sources can still fall through over time.

As an example of this, in the 2010's we had a contract with Molina Health in New Mexico. We had we set up numerous trainings and interventions at community health centers in rural New Mexico. We put months of effort into the project and it was getting off the ground. Then Molina lost the State of New Mexico contract for Medicaid, exited the state and the funding for that implementation died.

Without that money, the project was gone. Once you lose funding, no matter how good an idea you have, you're out of luck. I think that's part of the whole—I don't even know what to call it, maybe—journey. A lot of people don't understand about getting research into practice, or how to work that pipeline, and all of the different components that are required—all the different things that can go sideways.

At this point, I became aware of the work of Everett Rodgers, who was a researcher at the University of New Mexico and wrote the book, *Diffusion of Innovation*. His paradigm was most helpful to myself, and my research team and I highly recommend it to readers.

This brings us up to around 2013. We developed a moderate

drinking web application (moderatedrinking.com). A clinical trial demonstrated its efficiency. And then we came up with Overcomingaddictions.net, which had an abstinence focus protocol. To evaluate this abstinence protocol, we collaborated with Smart Recovery. And with that came a grant to combine all these extant programs into what became Checkup and Choices.

When we put this together with other elements concerning potentially addictive substances, such as opioids and stimulants, we tapped into a pool, finding people with the most expertise in their respective areas, from a clinical research standpoint.

What we've found with long-term research, from participants in moderate drinking studies, is that many, many people who are successful with moderate drinking eventually stopped drinking.

And that's harm reduction to the max.

Most people who do change their drinking do so on their own without ever going to professional treatment. Once they decide that the consequences of what they're doing are unacceptable to them to varying extents, they make those decisions themselves. And in the end that's the good news.

Reid can be reached at reidkhester@gmail.com

ADI JAFFE

I earned my PhD at UCLA but had no classes on harm reduction. The term wasn't even mentioned—the words "harm reduction" were not even spoken in a single class I took. We worked from a very NIDA-informed medical model. Addiction is a brain disease. It's a chronic illness. There is no cure. The best you can do is abstain forever. I drank the Kool-Aid fully. When I graduated, I was very much an "addiction is neuroscience-based" believer, which meant I put most of my hope for recovery in medication or medical procedures.

Ironically, my own story was not one of abstinence. This was in 2003. So more than twenty years ago now. I was about three years into my version of recovery. I'd stopped meth but had started drinking again. I was learning about the biology behind this at UCLA a couple of years later. There's a gap between my experience and what I learned about addiction and treatment, and the understanding of exactly *how* those two function together. At UCLA, we studied cognitive behavioral therapy, and I learned a little bit about motivational interviewing principals, contingency management, all the peripherals that go with that.

I just got to this place where my experience and what I was learning at school about addiction were not aligning.

By the time I started my postdoc, I conducted a study on why people don't get into treatment, or why they don't stay in treatment. One of the main barriers we found was abstinence. People don't want to abstain. And when I presented on that, the answer I would always get was, "Well, those people aren't serious about stopping their addiction." I'd challenge my professors. I'd ask, "Why do you say that?" Their responses were knee-jerk. I was trying to look at this scientifically. First of all, we had no measure for how "serious" somebody was—that was an abstract measurement based on personal biases on the part of the research team! At least, you shouldn't make conjectures about what someone is thinking, which you can't possibly know. But the other piece was, we only had about sixty people participate in the study, a six-month, basic examination of people who were actively looking for treatment. We had an online treatment finder. So I'd ask my professors and others espousing 12 Step programs, "Why would you say this person is not interested in getting help when the only way they found us was by *looking* for help?" That seems counterintuitive. If you see somebody walking out of the store with bread, it would be a stretch to say, "that person probably doesn't like bread." It wouldn't make sense.

That's when I really first started coming to terms with the fact that maybe the way I'd been taught wasn't all there was to the story. I began reaching out to experts in the field, who exposed me to other ideas, including harm reduction.

I finished my PhD in 2010, and then I started teaching. I was teaching a lot of addiction-related classes. I taught at Cal State

Long Beach, and I was using what I'll just call a more realistic, "real-world" approach to the subject of substance use. I think that's really where I learned the most about harm reduction and its application: from talking to college students.

I wasn't going to make the stupid mistake of saying you shouldn't drink and use drugs, because that's like telling a four-year-old they shouldn't play and take risks. That age is all *about* experimentation. Just say no. Sure, sound advice. But it's not reality. I began teaching some of the concepts from harm reduction. The more I taught it, the more comfortable I became with this idea of abstinence not being for everyone. Never mind that I was fully practicing it myself.

I ended up opening an outpatient treatment center with my partner at the time. One of our main distinguishing factors was that we were not abstinence-only based. If people wanted to learn how to moderate or if they wanted to learn how to take breaks, or slow down, whatever they wanted to learn, we were there to help them get there.

The originating concept of therapy is a harm reduction model. We're going to try to reduce your pain, your harm, and take care of you. It's only when we apply these same principles to recovery and addiction that it becomes problematic. Structured treatment programs have a really hard time with non-abstinence. We were trying to break that. We had a lot of uptake working for us. If I'd known how to run a business better, we probably would still be around and be more successful. But it was my first business and I was learning on the job. It was tough, running a program that challenged the 12 Step institution. We'd get hate phone calls, threatening emails telling us we're crazy and that we're gonna kill people. It was intense.

On one level, I get the fear. Obviously, the answer to stopping all opioid overdose deaths is for people to never use opiates. It's just not realistic. That approach has been failing us for decades. Not to mention, the drug serves a useful purpose, which is why medications like morphine were invented. There's another casualty in the War on Drugs, and we're seeing it right now with chronic pain patients, who get caught in the crosshairs. Opioids are a great example because people can get addicted to opiates and become physiologically dependent with or without a trauma, predisposed personality, history, genetics, etc. Opioids do have a strong physiological grip in a way. Some people need them to manage chronic pain. The vast majority of people who get addicted—and want to later get off them—will need support that extends far beyond the physiological dependence. Part of the problem with the abstinence-only model, in my opinion, is that it sometimes puts the cart before the horse. It suggests or purports that if we take care of the issue of the drug use first, then everything else will fall in place. Sometimes, maybe. But more often whatever underlying issue there is—whether that's chronic pain or psychological trauma—will remain after the drug use stops unless it's addressed.

I've had to learn how to speak and walk a fine line. Because I'm not advocating for moderation. And I'm not against abstinence. I'm for helping people. I'm for whatever is the most effective, efficient, and realistic way to help them. So *any* positive change is a *good* change.

Adi Jaffe can be reached through his website at https://www.adijaffe.com

SCOTT KELLOGG

have been, and I continue to be, horrified by the disastrous impact of addictions on the mind, body, spirit, freedom, and beauty of human beings. This distress has been a driving force in my work as an addiction psychologist, as a harm reduction psychotherapist, and as a Chairwork psychotherapist.

In the face of this, I have been centrally focused on three overlapping questions: How do people change, heal, and transform their lives? What are the psychological and psychosocial *mechanisms of change* that are involved? and how can I utilize them in my psychotherapeutic work? In my efforts to answer these questions, I have had deep encounters with many different forms of healing and psychotherapy; I have also had the opportunity and the great privilege of being able to take part in a series of collaborations with my friend and colleague, Andrew Tatarsky, the creator of Integrative Harm Reduction Psychotherapy. The outcome has been my efforts to integrate the wisdom of harm reduction psychotherapy with my practice of Chairwork psychotherapy.

Historically, harm reduction psychotherapy was a sea change in our understanding and treatment of people wrestling with addictions or problematic substance use. Some of its benefits are:

It means that therapists can simply love their patients[1].

Clinicians can be more relaxed as they no longer need to take the stance that they know what is right for their patients; instead, they can work with them and collaborate on the creation of goals and the strategies needed to attain them.

It accepts that while some patients will make rapid and dramatic changes, others will want to engage in a process of gradual change; "any positive change" is accepted as a form of progress and success.

It was the first psychotherapy that effectively understood that many patients will need to work on their addictive behavior and on the psychological and emotional pain and anguish that underlie and drive these behaviors in an integrated and empowering manner. It embraced the idea that experiences of trauma and self-hatred may need to be addressed before the patient will be willing to engage with their substance use issues.

---

1 Most Harm Reductionists reject the use of the term "patient"—preferring terms like "client" or "people who use drugs" instead. I believe that this is rooted a desire to challenge the power or "expertise" differential that has traditionally existed in psychotherapy and addiction treatment settings; I think that it also reflects a movement to de-pathologize substance use itself. While I resonate with these concerns, I also believe that the deep suffering and profound devastation that is a central and defining part of the addiction journey is, ironically, often trivialized. It is for this reason that I use the term "patient;" it is my way of acknowledging the profundity of the experience and my deep respect for them as individuals.

It understands that long-term recovery—whether involving drug use stabilization, moderation, nonaddictive use, or abstinence—is built on the creation of meaningful and rewarding identities that will conflict with and replace those that are based on the addictive use of substances.

Harm Reduction Psychotherapy, like other forms of psychotherapy, places a central emphasis on developing a strong therapeutic relationship with each patient. Erich Fromm, in *The Art of Loving*, defined Love as "the active concern for the life and growth of that which you love." I think this is a very good stance for a therapist to take toward their patients.

In turn, many patients who are addicted or who have a problematic relationship with substances, are living with a great deal of pain—pain that has often been there for a long time. This suffering may have roots in their personal histories, it may be related to their being members of historically oppressed or marginalized communities, or some combination of the two. Substance use, then, can be understood as a way of coping, as a kind of personal medicine, to help them survive in the world. One of the problems, however, is that this way of coping has become "unmoored"—to use a term from the work of Patt Denning and Jeannie Little—and has taken on a life of its own. This means that the therapy will challenge both the patient and the therapist to be able to flow back and forth between the underlying suffering, on the one hand, and the challenge of managing any ongoing substance use to minimize its harm and danger—as best as possible.

Chairwork was originally created by Jacob Moreno as a part of

Psychodrama, and it was adopted and re-envisioned by Frederich "Fritz" Perls, the creator of Gestalt Therapy in the 1960s; it has since been adapted and re-envisioned by psychotherapists from many different traditions. I discovered the extraordinary beauty and power of Chairwork in 2001, and I fell in love with it. An elegant, flexible, and powerful method of healing, it has been the central focus of my therapy practice ever since.

Chairwork is fundamentally based on multiplicity of self or the understanding that all people contain what has variously been called different parts, modes, voices, or selves within them, and that each of the parts has their own history, roles, and messages. While most of these parts have good intentions, others are internalizations of abusive figures that live inside the person with malevolent intent. While the parts of most people are somewhat out of balance, in psychopathological states, such as depression, anxiety disorders, traumatic reactions, personality disorders, and addictions, there is a much greater degree of imbalance. Given that, the "True North" of the psychotherapy process is to help strengthen the part of the self that Freud called the ego and what Chairwork psychotherapists call the "Inner Leader." As this part gets stronger, the individual will: (a) grow in their capacity to engage in emotional self-regulation by becoming better able to tolerate and successfully manage painful emotions and stress; (b) have better and more successful relationships with other people; and (c) be able to lead a self-directed life—a value-based life that is meaningful, assertive, and effective. What I find to be strikingly synergistic about this is that as the Inner Leader gains in strength and power, the patient will begin to regain their freedom, and their substance use will become more regulated, the inner storms related to trauma and self-hatred will start to abate, and problematic interpersonal and coping behaviors— such as passivity, rage, aggression, dissociation, and grandiosity—will lessen as well. Again, this is why I see the ongoing development of the Inner Leader as the "True North" of the therapeutic process.

In terms of the actual clinical work, Chairwork psychotherapy generally takes three forms. In the first, the patient sits in one chair and imagines someone from their past, present, or future in the chair opposite and talks to them. This could be a deceased grandfather, a partner or spouse, or an unborn child; this dialogue is often used when there is "unfinished business" or unresolved issues with other people. In the second, the patient moves to another chair and shares, in part or in whole, difficult or traumatic stories and memories. In the third, the patient moves to different chairs to: (a) give voice to different parts, and (b) create dialogues between these parts and the Inner Leader. Each of these can be used as forces of healing within the harm reduction psychotherapy framework.

For example, ambivalence—or mixed feelings about the use of substances—is often at the heart of the addictive experience. Using the Multiplicity of Self model, this can usefully be reframed as a conflict between two parts. Building on this, a Chairwork encounter can be created between these two parts. For example, using an imaginary patient named Harper, I would begin by working with Harper to make a list of the positives of continuing to use ("Continue") and the positives of making some kind of change ("Change")—however defined. The Continue side often affirms that the substances provide them with pleasure while also helping them to decrease pain and suffering; the Change side will often include anxiety about what the substances are currently doing to them and taking from them; they may also express a desire for a different and a better life.

To begin the Chairwork, Harper would be invited to move to Center or the Inner Leader chair. In this dialogue structure, there would be two chairs in front of them facing each other. Harper would then decide which chair would embody Continue and which would embody Change. Given that it is often useful to start with the status quo, Harper could go to the Continue chair and speak the truth of that part: "I want to keep using. I am hurting. I do not see how I would function without the drugs. I do not want to make any changes right now. I am not ready." They would then move the Change chair and embody that perspective: "I am not ready to stop either, but this is not working. I am scared; there must be a better way." The idea is for Harper to go back and forth five or so times—giving voice to each perspective as powerfully and as emotionally as possible. I often invite them to stand behind each chair as this would enable them to speak with greater authority and power.

After this is done, Harper would return to Center or the Inner Leader chair and be invited to feel the impact of the dialogue. It can be helpful for them to assess the relative weight of the two parts: e.g., 50:50, 60:40; 90:10, etc. Having taken in this information, Harper can then decide what if anything they would like to do. This could include taking no action while continuing the conversation, monitoring the experience more closely, engaging in some kind of substance use management, or moving to a more formal moderation structure. This work is clearly aligned with the values of harm reduction psychotherapy; while the therapist strives to create an emotionally compelling and intense encounter, the patient retains the freedom and ability to make an emotionally informed decision as to their next step or course of action.

As Andrew Tatarsky has affirmed, Harm Reduction Psychotherapy is a trauma-centered therapy, and Chairwork can be very useful in working through traumatic experiences. With a patient who wants to therapeutically engage with a difficult experience from the past, I would begin by having them sit in Center or the Inner Leader chair. They would then be invited to move to another chair and to tell a difficult story, a troubling memory, or a fragment of a memory in the *third person*. For example, if Harper had been in a car accident, they would be asked to tell the story of their car accident in the *third person*: "Harper was in a car accident, and these are some of the things that happened to them" rather than in the *first person*: "I was in a car accident, and these are some of the things that happened to me." After they told the story the first time, I would encourage them to stand up, move around, shake it off, and sit down and tell the story again. We would go through this process three or four times. What is striking about this process is that more details often emerge with each iteration; this is a sign that integration is taking place — which means that the person is beginning to heal. The *third person* approach is also helpful because it allows the patient to get more space from the trauma—which can make it less overwhelming and easier to tell. In the world of addiction and problematic substance use, many trauma stories are quite complex and tragic, and patients may feel deeply responsible for some of the things that happened and great shame about some of their actions; the *third person* storytelling method can help reduce these feelings and make these difficult narratives easier to approach.

As a next step, I would invite Harper to return to Center, and I would put several chairs in front of them. Depending on the specific details of their history, these chairs could represent and embody people who hurt them, people who knew that they were being mistreated and did nothing to protect them, and their younger self—the self that was the victim of the abuse. Harper would be encouraged to express his anger, fear, grief, and love—as appropriate—to each of these people. This can be a very powerful experience as many people have never had an opportunity to express these thoughts and feelings. Of note, it is not uncommon for those who went through childhood abuse to have difficulty expressing love, care, and compassion for their child self. When this happens, it is important that the therapist step in and speak directly to the child self-acknowledging what they went through with care, affirmation, and compassion. It can be a profound and healing experience for patients to hear other people talk about them in this way.

The experience of addiction is often filled with regret about past decisions and past actions—which may not only be a source of deep pain, but also an impediment to reclaiming and transforming one's life. If this were the case with Harper, I would first clarify the specific circumstances that they are upset about and the age that they were when these occurred. Adapting Tian Dayton's *Life Cycle Role Reversal* model, I would then invite them to sit in Center—in the Inner Leader chair—and imagine their younger self in the chair opposite. They would first be invited to speak to their younger self and give voice to the distress that they are feeling about what happened in the past. I would then ask Harper to switch chairs, to do a *role reversal*, and "become" their younger self. I would then interview this younger self to get their understanding of what they were going through at the time and how those decisions made sense to them. It is important that this work be done in an investigative manner—with the goal of seeking to understand rather than to be confrontational or critical. When this feels complete, I would ask Harper to move back to Center, to take a minute to let what the younger self said touch them, and then tell the younger self what they heard them say about the situations and challenges that they were facing. I would seek to encourage Harper to express compassion for their younger self. In general, I repeatedly emphasize the tragic nature of the addiction journey—a journey which leads many good people, under the influence of drugs or the compulsion of addiction, to do things that they find to be morally reprehensible—things that they never thought that they could or would do. Louise Hay, in *The Power Within You*, wrote: "There is no reason to beat yourself up because you didn't do better. You did the best you knew how." Similarly, Maya Angelou said: "You did what you knew how to do, and when you knew better, you did better." This is a challenging yet fundamentally healing perspective, and it is the spirit that I seek to embody in myself and cultivate in my patients.

While it is clear that Chairwork psychotherapy can be a profoundly transformative experience, we are still left with the questions: How does Chairwork work? How does it help people heal and transform their lives? I think that there may be three core factors. The first is *externalization* or the process of taking internal processes and putting them outside of the self so that they can be observed and engaged with. The second is that Chairwork involves the dimension of space which allows for creative and meaningful encounters between different parts of the self. The last is that the high levels of emotional arousal and intensity facilitate the resolution of traumatic experiences and the rebalancing of inner parts.

Harm reduction psychotherapy is, for me, a profoundly humanistic and compelling framework for working with patients who are wrestling with addictions or problematic substance use. Chairwork psychotherapy, in turn, is one of the more powerful and flexible forms of psychotherapy. The parts model can provide great therapeutic clarity as to the forces at work within the individual, and the emotional intensity of the dialogues can help patients not only work through past traumas, but also rebalance the forces within them. It is my hope that this work will spread and bring liberation to those who are trapped in the prison of addiction.

Scott can be reached at kelloggchairwork@gmail.com https://www.chairworkpsychotherapy.com

GARY LANGIS

I started working in harm reduction by accident really. Back in the early to mid-1980's, HIV was prevalent in my neighborhood. My late wife was HIV positive, and I had lost a lot of friends to the disease. I was seeing the damage caused by it, especially to IV drug users. I had stopped using heroin in 1972 so I could raise a family, get a job. And I did that. I got jobs. I started a business. I raised my family the best I could. And then I was injured on the job, a labor-intensive position. That was in the early 1980's and I was put on pain meds and one thing led to another and pretty soon I was taking them like candy. Before long I was strung out and on dope (heroin) again.

I was using down around the South End in Boston and would go down to the Boston City Hospital area to get heroin, to be around "us." And one of the users down there must have been a hospital attendant or something. He caught me using one day and started talking to me, asking if I used clean syringes, and I said, "I use what I can get." After that he started giving me new syringes. He asked, "Do you want to take some of these back to your friends?" I said, "Sure," so I started doing that secondary needle exchange. I didn't know what I was doing was harm reduction because, you know, there was no name for it yet. It was just me handing out new syringes given to me for other people to use so they wouldn't get infected with HIV and other diseases. And you know what? I started feeling good about doing it—this secondary syringe exchange, and then I started feeling good about myself. And that was a pretty new feeling.

After that experience, I started volunteering with an organized group of people doing HIV prevention, and one thing led to another and I just kept on. I still needed a job though, and began applying for positions. I couldn't go back to my main job because I had gotten badly injured the last time. It was an all-labor job and I couldn't do it anymore. I volunteered for a while until a job came open. It was an outreach worker position as an attendant in some recovery home. Then I saw this posting for a job working with folks with HIV. I got the job doing case management for people with HIV who used substances and needed to access disability benefits. I helped them to get Social Security, SSI benefits. About a year later, I became the program manager for that program. We worked in about five welfare offices throughout the Boston area, hooking people up with Social Security. We did really well. Our job was hard too. We were supposed to cut through the red tape of Social Security to help folks get access to disability benefits. It wasn't easy back then but it's even harder today.

It's funny because to get through the bureaucracy of the Social Security office, I used my past experiences networking with drug dealers and drug users since that world is really just another bureaucracy. On the case management job, we had to pick a number and stand in line for folks at various offices. We'd complete their application and then submit it. That helped us build a relationship with different folks in these offices where we were going daily. Eventually they were telling us to just come to the back door and bring the paperwork to them there. Oh my gosh! They even said, "Here, here's the code to get in the back door." Well that all stopped after the Oklahoma City bombing.

On the job, we kept going to the various offices, making friends with the office staff while putting in all these applications. We also helped when applications came up for reconsideration since there must be a person to represent the applicant before an administrative law judge. We did it all and we got about eight hundred people or more on Social Security benefits. It was really beneficial to them. I wound up working specifically with our homeless population for years. And then, in 1982, they started the Big Dig in Boston and that disrupted everything.

I left that case management job because the grant was running out. Then I got a job up on the North Shore and became the HIV program manager at some big treatment agency. Part of my job there was to integrate harm reduction into our treatment agency. The outreach program was providing education outreach and the agency hoped that we could help some of the drug users. That was probably my first official paying job in harm reduction. I stayed at that position for about 13 years.

When I left that agency, I went to work for the Education Development Center in Waltham. They were a large international organization, and we would collaborate with coalitions that were working on substance use prevention, as well as working to prevent fatal and non-fatal overdoses. I worked there for quite a long time. Finally, I went over to BMC (Boston Medical Center).

There I found a fairly workable coalition that were choosing different strategies to reach drug users—and they all had their own ways of working. To reach drug users in the area, they wanted to use people with lived experience but people who were no longer using drugs, mainly a lot of recovery coaches. Well, that didn't turn out well since, as we all know, that's not the way to reach *current* drug users, especially in a harm reduction frame. These recovery coaches were folks who were interested in helping drug users into treatment and recovery, or at least they wanted to help folks who wanted to make a change. They were providing education, but their idea of education was to offer and promote abstinence-only recovery education. Those folks aren't the peers of current drug users; those are the peers of people seeking treatment, recovery. It became a real issue. I felt—and *still* feel—that folks should just stay in their lane, do their thing how they define recovery and if I need to refer someone who's ready to make a change, then I'd happily refer them to these coaches. I would hope they'd do same thing—if they had a drug user whose drug use was in the precontemplation stage, who aren't ready to make a change, I wanted them to send that drug user to a harm reduction organization, like a syringe exchange. That's where they should go, not somewhere that would try to force them into some meeting where they're really not welcome, because they can feel that right away.

We thought we were really making some inroads with our treatment agency's harm reduction efforts, and in some ways we were. But this work—and this is the worst part of it—it takes years to get anything finished. Grants, other funding, and now the opiate settlement funds. Everybody's an expert; everyone thinks they know how to best spend the money and especially what it means to do harm reduction. Too many people in this sphere are just saying the words, "We'll meet you where you're at if you're using drugs." What they really mean is, "You need to get where *we're* at and then we'll help guide you to recovery," which of course means abstinence most of the time. And with drug users, it just doesn't work that way. You have to embrace people who use drugs. You have to build *relationships* with them. So, I decided to just work for myself. I couldn't take it in those systems anymore.

When I started to do the secondary syringe exchange, I felt better about myself; I wanted to do more, to be better. And the same thing happens when people who use drugs start to do things like distribute Narcan to their peers. They feel good about that so they want to do more. Maybe they start teaching their peers how to use Narcan or something like that. And you know what? Those are the folks who are the absolute best at doing outreach work. That's *their* community. To me, that's what harm reduction is: creating spaces for drug users to do their thing, to get connected with each other. It's about creating a space for *drug users* to do harm reduction. It's not about someone else's agenda, what they have for you or want for you. That doesn't work. No change works that way—especially when you're talking harm reduction.

Harm reduction is many smaller things. In a situation where you get an infection or a disease where you can overdose, harm reduction is all about strategizing ways to (literally) reduce the harm of that disease or infection, like strategies working on a clean or safe drug supply. Right now, drug users don't have a choice. They may want to use heroin but there's no heroin out there anywhere these days. They don't have a choice. They have to use whatever is available. Boy, how different things would be if we had a safe drug supply! I know I've said many times and in many places, "Listen, if you really want to reduce fatal overdoses, you've got to reintroduce heroin back into the drug market." What is available right now is really dangerous stuff.

The only chance I see of changing things like the drug market is with harm reduction. I want to see drug users—current users—sitting at the policy tables and not just being stroked like they are now. The Feds have given lots of money to lots of people but they should really listen to some of the people that have been doing the work for over thirty years, and not bring in people who've fought the worth of drug users for decades, like treatment providers. We were all the antichrist to those providers; they hated us. Everything we did was "enabling" and "damaging," causing more drug use. But drug users don't need our encouragement to continue to use. They do that already all by themselves.

Hey, I'm from the old days of harm reduction, where we really used to connect because we had nobody else, so you'd go to national conferences and get together with people like you: drug users and harm reductionists. We all knew each other, and now there's just so many people out there saying that they're doing harm reduction. But you know what? Just giving syringes out? That's not harm reduction. That's one strategy, sure—and a good one. But building connections with drug users, creating that space where *they* can take leadership roles in the field, is really where harm reduction needs to make some inroads. We had a little bit of that at the beginning. I used to know quite a few directors of programs that used drugs, but they've died or they got pushed out. We've lost a lot of good people. It's brutal out there now.

I really wish folks would understand that harm reduction is not enabling people to use drugs. We're trying to reduce the dangers of using illicit drugs, the consequences of using them, so someone won't go to jail for the possession of heroin—life-changing things like that. And these really are life-changing events. And they affect users negatively. We're trying to prevent events like this from happening. Harm reduction isn't just giving people supplies to get high with. It's much more. We're trying to save lives out there! We're working on the chaos that takes place in a user's life. A lot of that chaos is *not* created by them but rather it's created by the systems of care, of incarceration, of treatment. Today it seems like there's just so much crap out there about harm reduction and we're trying to get the real information (to the public), what it is and all. The only way to do that is to see harm reduction recognized on its own. [Harm reductions) needs to start or create [its] own groups, and not be connected to some treatment agency or big organization. In our needle exchanges, we never had anybody's funding, received nobody's help. Instead, we all had to learn how to survive, together, just like drug users do. And we distributed more syringes than the state-funded programs, the SSPs. We reached a lot of people, and we used a lot of peers, and we paid peers—we literally gave them money, not a dumb gift card. That's the way it should be. I'd like to see more of this going forward.

The last thing I'll say is that I'm looking at a lot of peer involvement now, people who use drugs, not (employing) recovery coaches like we used before. We just have to find ways to pay them because a lot of the funders have a hard time giving drug users money. They believe that if you give a drug user money, they'll just go use it on drugs. But here's what really happens.

I had one participant tell me they bought a pair of sunglasses with the money they earned. "And that made me feel good, you know?" they told me. So just like I learned when I started handing out clean syringes: when you start to feel better about yourself, you start wanting to feel better again, in a different way—and you want to start to give back to your community more. I sure didn't think my experience was going to lead to where it did for me. But it did. And no one is more surprised than I am that things turned out pretty damn well for me and for many in my community.

Note: Gary and colleagues also founded the New England Prevention Alliance (NEPA) around 1996–97. Much harm reduction work around needle exchange and more was done under this banner, often still conducted underground.

Gary can be reached at garylangis@yahoo.com

BARRY LESSIN

I was working as a psychologist in a private practice specializing in substance-use disorders for over 30 years and in the mid-2000s was questioning the value of the work that I was doing and wondering how long I could continue working in the field. I was contemplating the end of my career and thinking about what I would be wanting to do.

Around this time, I was profoundly affected by a couple of significant events—one personal and one professional. My brother turned to me for help with my nephew who was struggling with mental health issues and substance use, and using my traditional one-size-fits-all abstinence-only approach, I educated them about the need for them to use a "tough love" approach and create some hard boundaries that would require my nephew to attend residential rehab and follow treatment and recovery recommendations or else they should not be in communication with him unless he was actively working in a program of recovery, abstinence.

My "expert" recommendations ended up being disastrous. About a year and a half later we got a call from a trauma center in Florida that he had a severe suicide attempt after his admission and discharge AMA (against medical advice). When we went down to visit him it was clear to me within five minutes of talking to him that he had a severe bipolar disorder, which had never been treated. Despite my brother having the resources to send him to the best rehabs in the country, the traditional treatment industry failed my family miserably and almost lethally. We eventually found an excellent residential psychiatric facility specializing in co-occurring disorders and my family is now extremely grateful and proud of my nephew for following through on all his treatment recommendations (which were aligned with his actual mental health and substance use concerns) and he has been in a stable period of well-being since then.

The next influence was professional when my clients started to die from overdoses and I didn't have any answers with my traditional treatment model. At the time I had created a new website and was looking for content. When I Googled various topics about addiction, I came across an article from the Drug Policy Alliance commemorating the 40th anniversary of the War on Drugs. Reading the article transformed my thinking. I began to view addiction through a public health lens and saw that the War on Drugs is a war on people and on families. I began reading as much as I could about people working in the harm reduction field. I read Dee-Dee's book and Gabor Mate's book *In the Realm of Hungry Ghosts*. Patt Denning and Jeannie Little's book *Over the Influence* was a harm reduction bible for me. It was inspirational reading about the harm reduction pioneers who were trained in similar ways I was but were using harm reduction approaches to impact clients in truly effective ways.

Social media allowed me to connect with some of the existing harm reduction community and I eventually met people and advocates like Gretchen Burns, Denise Cullen, and Julia Negron, who were working with families that had lost their kids or were struggling because their kids were struggling with their own addictions. They willingly and graciously invited me into their communities but there was a lot of pushback from the families in the community to someone like me—the psychologist coming into the mix was like the "enemy" entering the room. I realized that I represented the "treatment industry" that had failed them, and it was understandable that they were so angry and upset because they had lost so much. But they soon learned that I was someone who was willing to be open and I wanted to learn. I'm so grateful that they eventually embraced me as part of their community.

I was able to reach out professionally to harm reductionists Stanton Peele, Tom Horvath, Andrew Tatarsky, Sheila Vakharia, Scott Kellogg, and many others. They took time to speak with me, encouraged me, and invited me into this professional harm reduction community. Even though I had been working as a psychologist in the Philly suburbs for decades, was well known with an established practice, and had been to many conferences with colleagues, I never really felt like I was part of the traditional treatment community. I felt now that I wanted to be a part of this other community, this community of harm reductionists. There was something there that was very, very special and very different from my usual work.

My initial work in the drug policy advocacy world was with families who had lost loved ones to overdose and who were abandoned by the treatment industry. It was very painful and infuriating to watch and it made me really question what I had been involved in for over 30 years. I realized that I had to make some changes in my clinical work, to learn about harm reduction to find new ways of working with families. It also forced me to look at my own stigma and judgments about addiction and about those who use drugs. The stigma and judgments were so ingrained, it took me years—literally years—before I was able to let go of the drug war narratives about substance users. I realized that I was one of those people who judged and stigmatized drug users; who believed that they lied, cheated, and weren't ever honest with me.

For about five years, from 2011 to 2016, my advocacy work centered on educating families to empower them—thousands of them nationwide—to go into their communities to do grassroots work to help pass life-saving legislation. In 2014, I worked with a Pennsylvania group that helped the naloxone access and Good Samaritan bills get passed. These bills required that naloxone, the lifesaving opiate antidote, be accessible to more people who needed it. The 911 Good Samaritan Bill protected people from arrest if they called 911 during an overdose while trying to help someone who was overdosing.

Unfortunately, in the past few years it appears that drug policy advocacy and harm reduction work nationwide has stalled somewhat. It's apparent that the stigma against harm reduction is still very strong. We've spent so much time and energy educating people and giving them information about substance use and harm reduction, but they are bombarded with well-funded misinformation and agendas against this work. It became increasingly frustrating to try to move things forward from the progress we made. At times it felt like one step forward and two steps back. In the mid- to late-2010s, I decided to leave the advocacy side to focus on my harm reduction psychotherapy practice.

This year (2023), my itch to do more than clinical work found me connecting with Dr. Amanda Reiman, a PhD social worker and social scientist who's done a lot of research into the intersectionality of cannabis use and society. We're in the process of writing a textbook with the working title *Harm Reduction Approaches for Working with Substance Using Adolescents*. The book targets master's level psychology, counseling, and social work students to give them better skills in working with substance using adolescents and their families. I see my work on this textbook as similar to the advocacy work I did with families—it's like planting seeds, this time sharing my harm reduction knowledge with the next generation of students, similar to what we did with the parents and families in advocacy. The textbook will also help to further harm reduction education which is virtually non-existent in our graduate schools.

Since I began practicing harm reduction psychotherapy with adolescents, young adults and their families about twelve years ago, I can count on maybe two hands the number of people that I've needed to refer to residential care. This is because I'm offering them skilled individual- and family-centered treatment based on scientifically proven therapeutic methods such as cognitive behavior therapy, motivational enhancement, and DBT (dialectical behavioral therapy) skills training. I used to dread when a client would begin using drugs again and I thought, "What am I going to do now?" That's not even an issue anymore because I know that I can use the skills that I have learned as a harm reductionist, and the work I do has become a joy for me. Becoming a harm reduction therapist wasn't something that I had to learn, per se, but I did have to unlearn some bad behaviors and attitudes and work through the stigma I had about drug users. When I did, I was able to feel much more competent helping people in a positive way.

Today, I don't think harm reduction is that complicated. I simply think about how I want to be treated when I receive care. I want to be treated with compassion and respect for my own uniqueness. I want science-based information. I want to make choices for myself. I want people to understand the struggles that I've had and some of my obstacles. Why aren't we doing this? Why are we doing this other treatment, the one we've been doing for decades that clearly is not working with most people who use substances or engage in other risky behaviors? I realize now that doing harm reduction work is itself empowering by helping people to make decisions for themselves—and that was what was lacking in traditional treatment. It comes back to the basic idea that people are going to engage in risky behaviors, and they have a right to make their own choices. We look to try to shift the behaviors from being riskier to helping them make safer, better choices.

For me, the bottom line of harm reduction work is about being able to trust yourself as a parent and/or as a clinician, to help people to gain empowerment, and just follow the science. There's a lot of good science-based information out there but to access it you must be pointed in the right direction and that's what I hope I do for the families that I work with.

Barry Lessin can be reached at https://www.barrylessin.com

ALBIE PARK

My coming to harm reduction was an evolution. Probably the first time that it really occurred to me that the typical "abstinence-only" system was questionable was when I was working at my first job in treatment, which was at a residential facility for people with HIV and AIDS before there were any meds to treat the disease. At the time, the belief was a positive diagnosis carried with it a six-month to a year life expectancy.

I can't remember this guy's name—let's call him "Henry." In his 30's, Henry was a gentle and reserved black man who'd been using heroin at that point for ten years or so. When he stopped using opiates, which helped numb him from both emotional and physical pain, he found he had three major "gifts" of recovery. The first was learning how bad the neuropathy in his legs had gotten; it made *just* walking extremely painful. The second being that his teeth were rotting in his head, making eating painful. Last, since opiates are constipating, he had not known he had uncontrollable diarrhea related to HIV. So he couldn't get more than, like, two blocks away from the house without shitting himself. These were the "gifts" of sobriety. One day, he had signed out. We had a rule: if they weren't back within ten minutes of their stated return time, we had to lock the door. This particular day, there was a vicious storm in San Francisco, one of those intense storms we don't get often. I remember going to the door, and I can still see my hand reaching for the lock, and hear it turning as I'm thinking, "I just locked the door on a man with full-blown AIDS in the middle of a thunderstorm." In the moment, I said to myself, "This is wrong." At the time, even though it registered as a dissonant thought, I was able to shelve it. I was still influenced by the thought that abstinence was the only valid path to recovery. I stayed in the field for a couple more years before I had to leave because the house closed.

So, I became a massage therapist, then taught massage. An old friend, Michael Siever, asked me to work for him as a counselor for the Stonewall Project (the first true harm reduction treatment program in San Francisco)—this was when he was first starting it. I knew Michael from working as an administrative assistant for a mental health program. Michael was the director of the substance use treatment program. This was in my mid-20's and it had been several years since we had worked together. When he first approached me to be a counselor at Stonewall, I said, "Oh, hell no. I'm not going in the trenches again." A year or so later, my husband, Randy, developed a clot after about a week after neck surgery. He literally dropped dead in front of me. It was impossible for me to do massage while so grief stricken and I found myself desperate for work. Michael ended up offering me a job as the project assistant. Unfortunately, I was really bad at it now! He fired me after my probation period, which I deserved (for a long time, he would argue that he didn't fire me. We would joke about it but I really sucked at the job).

In the beginning, Stonewall shared an office suite with a pretty hardcore abstinence only treatment program unironically called STOP (Stimulant Treatment Outpatient Program). My last day at Stonewall, they were having a staff meeting. After they were done, a friend I worked with at the residential program said she hoped I would not be mad (she knew about my "not going back into the trenches" sentiment) but she had just suggested they hire me as a counselor for a half-time position. I was interviewed and hired within a week—mostly based on my friend's recommendation and the fact they really needed someone who could hit the floor running. Michael asked me why I would not work for him at Stonewall in the same capacity. Now that I had gone back into the trenches, I had no excuses, so I finally took the half-time counselor position at Stonewall. STOP was a morning and afternoon program while Stonewall was in the afternoons and evenings. In the mornings I worked in a pretty typical "abstinence only" milieu and in the afternoons a pretty hard-core harm reduction setting.

Obviously, this set me up to compare and contrast the differing philosophies. What I found was harm reduction gave me a vast array of new tools to work with someone. As a provider, I realized that Stonewall offered people many more ways to explore what was going on. Unlike a typical abstinence focus, where the counselor is considered the expert [which] sets up an immediate hierarchy, harm reduction gave me the opportunity to be much more collaborative and curious. This allowed folks to be more honest with me.

When I first started in the field, the minimum requirement was to have a degree or to have two years of continuous sobriety, which I had at that time. I was an art major, which meant I was used to looking at the particular and the general together. I was able to capture both the nuance and the broader strokes of someone's story. Understanding things from this perspective was incredibly helpful and I found my work at Stonewall to be more effective by defining recovery and treatment as something that *might* or might not include abstinence. Understanding the Stages of Change[1] also helped the folks I worked with to be less judgmental and kinder to themselves. With the Stages of Change, I knew that when folks returned to their old behaviors, I needed to help them figure out what had happened. They often needed help figuring that out and I usually first heard "I don't know" when I asked, but I also explained that there's always a reason or a starting point, and that needed to be uncovered and unpacked. This was the work of treatment—seeing what works and what doesn't and what could work better.

Michael trained so many interns at Stonewall. I remember talking to him once and he told me he always waited for a new intern to come into his office for supervision and confess they had no idea what they were doing. That was when Michael would say, "Good. Then we can start working." As an art major I already knew in a sense I had no idea what I was doing and used to joke that I made shit up as I went along. What I mean is I stayed curious and respectful and really understood the concept of people being the experts in their own lives. This meant understanding my clients as individuals and working with them according to the nuances of their stories.

I stayed in harm reduction because I believe in this. At first, like many, I viewed harm reduction as a specific professional modality. I didn't yet understand that harm reduction has much broader implications. Harm reduction changed the way I look at and approach everything.

I had a very interesting conversation yesterday with my best friend, whose oldest son had been free from alcohol for a year and a half. Previously, she'd been a really hardcore 12 Step kind of mom—hook, line, sinker, tough love, codependency, all of it. She used to think what I did was a bit crazy. Over time and conversation, she started to change her stance, and that's when things really changed for her son. She said to me, "There's so much less pressure [with harm reduction]." She came to appreciate more flexibility in a person's progress rather than insistence on sobriety only. The "all or nothing" stance rules out anyone who doesn't succeed 100%. Harm reduction has forced me to re-learn basic ideas of relating to and communicating with others, and to respect people who do things I personally don't understand and might even describe as self-destructive.

I define harm reduction as a self-conscious decision to resist the temptation to dehumanize others and I admit to failing miserably at it sometimes! The short-hand version: *harm reduction is love*. In my professional capacity, I have to find a person's humanity and often what this really means is helping that someone re-discover their own.

I don't consider harm reduction a public-health issue. Public health policy tries to solve complex problems with broad strokes, providing systemic answers to those problems. I think this encourages the phenomenon of someone becoming their diagnosis, as opposed to being a person. People become things to fit into categories as opposed to being individuals. I like to believe we've influenced public health so much that we've taken on some of the unpacking of diagnosing, categorizing, and moving toward a more humanizing philosophy.

People get tired of being told what type of lives can be saved. I think the inherent limitations of public health—the ways in which harm reduction got rolled out via a public health model for obvious reasons—has also inherently created stumbling blocks. Too many people are dedicated to the idea of keeping harm reduction as public health period or primarily as public health. And I don't know if that's as productive long-term or as viable as people might think.

We also can't ignore the financial aspect. Harm reduction must figure out ways to help employ people who are unemployable because of felonious history. It bothers me that the community is so scattered. How do we generate unrestricted funds? What are our economic options? How is it that we can expand this way? For instance, each year, AIDS Lifecycle—a weeklong charity bike ride from San Francisco to LA—raises up to $15 million dollars for the AIDS Foundation and LA Gay and Lesbian Center. What if *we* were able to generate that much money? In order for harm reduction to reach its full potential, people need to understand its breadth beyond public health.

We need to reach people on emotional levels. How do we create mechanisms for people to share stories that are outside of the typical abstinence-only narrative? There's a misperception that [harm reduction] excuses bad behavior. That's not true. Harm reduction is about meeting people where they are, being respectful, and allowing room for difference.

We need to shed the mentality that only *one* way works. In fact, 28 days—the standard rehab stay—does *not* work. This is all about what insurance will pay for treatment. These programs are often confrontational. Some people respond well with that structure. Many more will bristle at the "do as I say or get the fuck out" approach. Sure, tough love might work sometimes. But we must be open to other avenues when it doesn't. We have to start treating each drug user as an individual. Otherwise, we might lose them before we or they get the chance to begin.

One of the reasons I started working in harm reduction was to help get the message out, partly because simply calling it "public health" is not enough. I also see the conflict between chronic pain and harm reduction, particularly some pain advocacy folks who feel those stupid drug addicts ruined it for everybody. That can't be where people are starting from. I would like harm reduction to break the bounds of public health, take it beyond substance use, so people experience and understand that being kind, loving, compassionate, respectful, humble—these are good places to start healing more than simply unwanted drug use or dependency. You have to care for people as people.

Lastly, I want to address the adage that harm reduction is part of abstinence, but abstinence is not necessarily a part of harm reduction. I firmly believe that harm reduction is a part of abstinence. On the way to achieving this lofty abstinence goal, many people have tried some harm reduction approaches without knowing it. Some go through a period of abstinence in order to figure out what the fuck is going on with them. Then they can say, "Okay, now that I've stepped back and taken stock of the situation, how do I want to reintroduce this to myself? Can I use again? Can I smoke pot or drink wine with dinner because I never had a problem with those?" In general, when asked these questions by clients or others, I answer that I don't know but it's their right to find out. Many people put abstinence and harm reduction in opposition. And they're absolutely not in opposition. In fact, from what I just said, I see them working in tandem. They can—and should—be supportive of each other.

Albie can be reached HRH413.org & harmreduction.works

Endnotes

1. The Stages of Change or Transtheoretical Model of the Stages of Change (TTM) were developed by James Prochaska, PhD & Carlo DiClemente, PhD in the late 1970's. The following is the original journal article from their research: Prochaska, J. O., & DiClemente, C. C. (1983). Stages and processes of self-change of smoking: Toward an integrative model of change. Journal of Consulting and Clinical Psychology, 51(3), 390-395. http://doi.org/10.1037/0022-006X.51.3.390.

GEORGE PARKS

For the past 30 years, I have been involved in harm reduction as a program developer and trainer. I have been fortunate in my career to have G. Alan Marlatt as my mentor, lifelong colleague and close friend. In clinical psychology research, Alan was a controversial figure in a newly emerging science-based understanding of addiction, called "addictive behaviors." Most pertinent to my focus here, Alan was also seen as an inspiration for the evolving harm reduction framework of policy and community-based programs that began emerging in the U.S.A. in the 1990s. He is considered by many to be the "founding father" of harm reduction therapy. As a student (and later colleague) of Marlatt, I came to harm reduction eagerly and excitedly at the beginning of efforts to develop harm reduction principles and practices as a form of psychotherapy.

What is harm reduction therapy? Rather than embracing the disease or moral model of alcoholism or addiction, harm reduction is a public-health approach to preventing and reducing the harm of alcohol or drugs that was born from the immediate needs, and in the collaboration with, people who use drugs in ways that harm themselves and others. HRT is both a client-centered and evidence-based approach founded on the philosophy of compassionate pragmatism. Compassion is expressed in empathy, acceptance, and understanding of the client; pragmatism is the development of psychotherapies that are evidence-based.

At the inception of HRT, Alan, our colleagues, and I were severely criticized by advocates of both the disease and moral models of addiction because HRT does not require abstinence as a goal; it accepts clients who are still drinking alcohol or using other drugs, and respects the autonomy and decision-making of the client as the guiding principle of therapy. Harm reduction therapy is an alternative to seeing addictive behaviors as diseases that create helpless victims who admit their powerlessness over alcohol or other drugs, adopt a stigmatized identity, commit to lifelong abstinence, embrace a "higher power," and enter and work the 12 Steps of recovery. Harm reduction therapy is also an alternative to the moral model of addiction expressed in the U.S. by the "War of Drugs." This model has caused a long history of judging and severely punishing people who use certain drugs due to character defects that promote addiction and anti-social behaviors. In 1996, the "War on Drugs" was raging and 30-years later (2024), the fact that harm reduction came to America (in the '90s) has changed the landscape of how we address people whose drug use causes harm to themselves and others. The "War on Drugs" goes on, but harm reduction policy advocates and organizations continue to promote a public health alternative to addressing the harm caused by alcohol and drug use.

Like a lot of people, my road to harm reduction comes from my lived experience of drug-related harm. My parents met after World War II. My dad was a PTSD veteran and my mom was a French-Canadian who only spoke French and was forced to emigrate to Columbus, Ohio, because of her pregnancy with me. They had me and three other kids in five years. They started drinking heavily, really heavily, and fighting nearly all the time: drinking and fighting. And my poor mother was taking diet pills—methamphetamine—while my dad was drinking cans of beer in the car while he delivered food. At 11 p.m. every night, my folks would get together after their long days to watch Johnny Carson and start fighting again. It was brutal, alcohol-fueled, stupid fighting that kept me awake all night. It really, really hurt me. So, my first experience with harm reduction was harm *induction*.

Alcohol is toxic, and it caused me to have severe trauma. Today I would be diagnosed with chronic PTSD, or childhood PTSD. My siblings just somehow armored themselves but I couldn't stop the toxic stuff from coming through. I responded with an oppositional defiant disorder, and started stealing from my parents and destroying property. I was arrested six times from eighteen to twenty. No one back then asked what was going on with me or what's happening at home. In spite of all the challenges, I was able to get into Ohio State University and avoid the draft. Then I joined the ROTC. I knew nothing about politics, just that ROTC was going to pay my way through my junior and senior year in college, and I thought I was going to Vietnam.

I eventually made the rank of second lieutenant. My friends that managed to return from Vietnam told me about their experiences over there, and they had all these drugs. I had never used any drugs (outside of alcohol). They had gum opium, they had Thai stick marijuana, they had psilocybin mushrooms. They also had keys of marijuana from Mexico. So when they came back, they totally radicalized me and I suddenly had access to all these good quality drugs. I quit ROTC. I became a hippie in the winter of 1970, just before the riots. But then one of my friends got killed and that changed everything for me—more drugs and insanity. When I came to, I left all those people behind, including my parents.

Serendipitously, I got hired as a work study student in social psychology research. I made an amazing transformation. I was able to actually create a real me that was pro-social. These folks in the lab cared for me and I got to meet world famous faculty there. One of them became my mentor and asked me if I was going to graduate school. I said no because I had such an inferiority complex and such a sense of being defective from my childhood experiences. But I went to the University of Washington, and I met and came to really like—love—Alan Marlatt; we became close friends and that friendship would last a very long time. He encouraged me to get my PhD and that's how I got involved in alcohol research and of course harm reduction, because of Alan.

I studied all of Alan's and his colleagues' work while I was doing this dissertation. I had lived experience regarding the harm of alcohol and drugs and that led to a passion. But when I started studying for my dissertation, I discovered, for the first time, I knew nothing about the *tools* people need to help reduce the harm of alcohol and other drugs. I didn't come from 12 Step or from the moral model; with what I learned in my dissertation studies, I eventually came from a social psychology research tradition that created a discipline, "Psychology with Addictive

Behaviors." It was just those maladaptive coping strategies that give you initial pleasure and delay the pain but don't ever solve the problem, because you never really address the problem. I discovered that Alan and his colleagues had completely rejected the moral model popular, which they saw as absolutely unhelpful to understanding drinking and drug use. The moral model was unsubstantiated, more folklore and superstition. They began to actually study the behavior of addiction, and then use the term *addiction*. They created a discipline, which is now very strong in research: a field called the "Psychology of Addictive Behaviors." Alcoholism, or AUD as we call it today, is not a disease. The alcoholic or addicted behaviors are also not moral; they're *learned behaviors*.

In the Addictive Behaviors Model, alcohol and drug use are seen as maladaptive coping strategies to manage pain and increase pleasure, but at enormous costs. Most people suffering harm from their alcohol or drug use will deny or minimize that there are costs to their behavior, as I did for years, but you can't continue to do what I did—drink and use drugs like I did—without pushing all the harms aside in your awareness so you can to do it all over again the next day. Yes, there's pain and harm in heavy drinking, but there's so much reward in it, too. For me, the rewards of heavy drinking were social approval, a reduction in pain, and a temporary increase in pleasure.

We did research in a new laboratory that Alan had built on the second floor of the psychology building, which he got some private funding for, called the "BAR Lab." BAR stood for the "Behavioral Alcohol Research Laboratory." There, we were able to demonstrate conclusively that heavy drinking males will drink heavily when they're paired with another heavy drinking male. That idea was really revolutionary at the time. I was able to demonstrate that when you pair a person with heavy drinking habits with a light drinking person, the heavy drinking person reduced their drinking. This was new thinking! And it's a good prevention message, especially for young adults. We could tell them that "once you get on campus and you get to the dorm, there's gonna be a lot of drinking, and there's gonna be a lot of heavy drinkers to hang with them, so you're gonna probably drink heavily too. But if you can find some way to hang out with the light drinkers, you're going to probably be a light drinker." In real life, light drinkers don't really affect the heavy drinkers because the two don't often hang out together. The other thing I demonstrated in that lab was that social anxiety increased drinking, no matter how much the other guy drank.

In our research on college drinking, our team developed a group-delivered harm reduction program called the Alcohol Skills Training Program (ASTP) that was a combination of motivational enhancement, alcohol harm prevention education, and coping skills training. This 8-week group reduced the peak drinking of participants from .14 BAC to .06 BAC, lowering the students' level or intoxication and reducing harms of drinking. The ASTP program was the first intervention developed that demonstrated to produce a reduction in college student drinking.

Encouraged by these results we replicated the ASTP in a 6-week group and decided to also develop and test a one-on-one harm prevention program modelled in part on a community-based brief intervention developed by Bill Miller called the "Drinker's Checkup," by using motivational interviewing and coping skills training as the treatment modalities. Our research team developed a similar program based on the content of ASTP and the structure of the

Drinker's Checkup, which came to be called BASICS (Brief Alcohol Screening and Intervention for College Students).

BASICS is a *Brief Motivational Intervention* (BMI) designed for selective or indicated alcohol harm prevention program in college students and other emerging adults who are engaging in episodic heavy drinking and have experienced, or are experiencing, alcohol-related problems. Following a harm reduction approach, *BASICS* aims to motivate students to make changes in their quantity and frequency of drinking in order to decrease the negative consequences of alcohol they and those around them were experiencing. I also developed CASICS (Cannabis Screening and Intervention for Collège Students) in 2014 and have included it my workshops even since. While today, BASICS and CASICS are a common services offered by most College Wellness Programs, what is also inspiring and gratifying to me is that harm reduction has become the dominant service delivery model for college prevention and health promotion programs throughout the county.

This all may not seem very important or groundbreaking but 30 years ago, there was no research on alcohol and drugs. In fact, Alan went to his hero, Albert Bandura, at Stanford—yes, the father of social learning theory—and Alan said, "Look, my friends at college are telling me not to do research on this, that it's gonna ruin my reputation." And Albert Bandura said, "Where do we need science more? In a place where people are hurting themselves and killing themselves, and where they have no evidence-based way to understand it all or be helped?" God bless him for that!

One of the things I love is this modern expression that the addiction is actually the *solution!*

Now of course we humans will deny that there is a cost to our behaviors with alcohol and other drugs. But you can't continue to do what I did—drink and use drugs like I did—without pushing aside all the harms to do it again the next day. Yes, there's pain but there's so much reward in it, too. There's so much social approval, and a reduction in pain, and a temporary increase in pleasure. Through all this what we discovered was that the psychology of addictive behaviors includes things that don't involve alcohol and drugs, that there are behavioral addictions like gambling. And of course that led to my buddy Stanton Peele and Archie Brodsky writing their book *Love and Addiction*. That book was also one of the first things Alan and I read, along with Andrew Weil's book, *The Natural Mind*.

All of this led to a lot of research in this new field. These were the people that got the money because they were doing rigorous, really good research. They discovered that a biopsychosocial model was much more evidence based because the research was also coming from medicine and psychotherapy. The way to understand addictive behavior, to address these behaviors we learned, is to use cognitive behavioral therapy or CBT. It was the mid-1970's and at that time everyone, including Bill Miller, was getting trained in CBT. It was even called *The Cognitive Revolution*.

Of course, this new approach was all dammed by psychologists even though it was done by people with a deep psychology approach. CBT was seen as trivial, and it was also seen as betrayal of the pure behaviorist (philosophy), which says thoughts don't matter. Well, Aaron Beck and a bunch of other folks within the addiction field like David Burns showed that CBT was important. And the other thing that happened at this time, which Alan and I found so powerful, was that instead of celebrating helplessness and loss of control like behaviorists, CBT celebrated *empowerment*. We said it gave power to the people.

Others called it self-management or self-control. It was an empowerment model, not a helplessness or disempowerment model. Our model for alcohol and other drug use didn't say things like "all you can do is never drink again." None of that "just go to meetings and work the steps." Our model said, "You're not powerless. You're not bound to this behavior. This behavior can be changed. Will it be easy? No, it will be really, really hard. And it will be painful because the only way beyond the pain is through the pain." It was remarkable. This was harm reduction even though we weren't calling it that yet.

The other thing that Alan was doing, along with studying the biopsychosocial aspects of addictive behaviors, was a study on the effects of aversion therapy on the relapses of recovering alcoholics. The thinking was that behavior therapy would shock those people to their senses. But it didn't work. In fact people had more relapses! This ultimately led Alan to study relapse prevention based on the sample of 54 people who relapsed: what happened, and how and where and when, and how did they feel? He developed a very thorough interview and studied every aspect of these relapses. He created a typology of what we now call "high risk situations." And then he did a prospective study, where he gave people questionnaires and asked them when they relapsed and which one of these factors was the most prominent. He found that 75% of their relapses were caused by interpersonal conflict, negative feelings and social pressure. Then he did some research, and Kathleen Carroll did some research, and it turned out that this "cognitive behavioral risk prevention model" turned into a therapy that was more effective than anything else we had, called "RPT." Alan asked me to create a RPT group program, therapy manual, and practitioner training. I did so, and delivered my RPT program practitioner training to substance abuse treatment centers and community corrections programs throughout the country.

The next thing that happened was really remarkable, just mind boggling. Up in Canada, there was the idea—just like with addictions—that criminal conduct was a disease or a moral failing. And nothing worked to rehabilitate people. Almost a parallel to America with addictions. There was a guy up there named Don Andrews, who was parallel to Alan, and his partner, John Bonta, who's parallel to me. And they created a cognitive behavioral social learning thing called "the psychology of criminal conduct." And the same way that Alan studied addictive behaviors, they reconceptualized criminal conduct as a *learned behavior*. And instead of saying nothing works, they set out to find what *does* work.

And the next thing you know, the Correctional Service of Canada, the Federal Bureau of Prisons in the United States, and several states searching for evidence-based approaches to behavior change wanted to implement cognitive behavioral relapse prevention, based on our RPT model. Most of the administrators of these corrections facilities would never have agreed to this RPT (Relapse Prevention Therapy) curriculum that I designed from our research if they knew it was harm reduction, so we never called it that. Despite federal laws concerning drug possession and use, not a single word in the RPT manual and client workbook requires abstinence. Consequences of relapse or recidivism were discussed, but not one was told what to do with that information. Instead, they were empowered to make their own best choice. So yeah, it's all harm reduction.

They implemented it and you know what they found out? The "Cognitive-Behavioral Relapse Prevention Model" developed into a therapy was more effective than any other approach in treatment of alcohol or other drug problems. They found reductions in relapse and reductions in recidivism in both systems, even in the American system. Reductions in recidivism. Too bad we didn't stick with it. This was the '90's and now we're in the 21st century. So much of this information and research has been unknown or lost and it's really a shame. In fact, I think it's immoral when you find something that can help people and you stop using it. But that's the way of the systems in which we live.

At this point I should probably define what I call harm reduction. Harm reduction is founded on the philosophy of *compassionate pragmatism*. This philosophy guides the development of policies, grounded in wellness and public health, that do not judge or punish people for possessing or using "illegal drugs." Compassionate pragmatism also encourages and supports the creation of programs like needle exchange, and all the other things that people who use drugs have been clamoring for the last 50 years. Harm reduction supports programs that serve the needs of people who use drugs, focusing on reducing the harm caused by their drug use, and improving their overall quality of life. These harm reduction programs are generated from a person's own assessment of what they want and need. Come as you are, we'll meet you there. Finally, harm reduction therapy (HRT) provides practices so that people [can] meet people where they are with acceptance, empathy, and understanding.

Harm reduction therapies are delivered by psychologists, mental health professionals, counselors, social workers and peers. These harm reduction therapy practices focus on improving the individual's coping strategies to reduce the harms of drug use.

Look, we're always going to be harm reductionists and, at some level, that makes us the loyal opposition. We are like "rebels with a cause." So many people are doing something new in the area of harm reduction and especially harm reduction therapy practices; it's great to see. I consider there to be three harm reduction therapy nodes: the Seattle node, focusing on research and program development along with the Addictive Behaviors Research Center; the San Francisco node, focusing on programs and community engagement and practices of harm reduction therapy with Jeannie Little and Patt Denning (until recently); and the New York mode, the integrated harm reduction psychotherapy (with) Andrew Tatarsky. What we need now is for the people who took over the San Francisco model to keep on keeping on. We currently have an HRT Research Center on UW campus with Alan's former postdoc students who have just written a book, *How to Do Harm Reduction Therapy*. I really want to see a radical change in policy like Oregon and Portugal have so that our country would have no illicit drugs; all drugs would be legal. And they would be regulated in fair, humane ways, not by the Drug Enforcement Administration. One of the things that really bugs me and that I worry about in the future is CRAFT, which is an attempt to get people into treatment without being abusive, and it does help them get into treatment, which could be good. But then I asked myself, what's the treatment like? A lot of treatment centers seem to be using more inclusive and even harm reduction language but generally they just know how to do process

328

groups. We really need to that improved. And we need to see cannabis legalized nationally. I want to continue to see harm reduction centers all over America, primarily programmatic to include needle exchange, safe injection sites, methadone, and all the other great things that the people who use drugs need. Those are my harm reduction dreams!

The last thing I want to share is my wish that despite the fact that we have for the most part stopped using words like abuse, alcoholic, junkie, pothead, etc., we haven't stopped using the words "drug user." And "drug user" is just as pejorative, just as stigmatizing, as the rest. I've seen a lot of people now calling others "people who use drugs," or PWUD. I want everywhere in this country to be a place where people are not defined by characteristics like drug use, sex, gender identity, sexual orientation, age, race, etc. I want to see us live in a place where people are people first, and their biological, psychological, and social characteristics are personal qualities, not identities or characteristics to be judged and punished for.

I want to see a humanistic future, one in which people do you no harm because of your alcohol or drug use and where people practice compassionate pragmatism to try to supportive and to be helpful to those who are suffering and in need our assistance. I believe harm reduction is ultimately, at its heart, an expression or radical love.

George can be reached at CompassionatePragmatism.com

Endnotes

1. Oregon just rescinded their recent attempt to decriminalize drugs.

2. CRAFT stands for Community Reinforcement Approach and Family Therapy developed by Robert Meyers, PhD. You can find more at robert-jmeyers.com or through the Center for Motivation and Change at www.motivationandchange.com

JEREMY PRILLWITZ

I got court mandated many years ago and was sentenced to go into treatment and to attend 12 Step meetings. I'm the kind of person who tries to make the most of a situation. That was my attitude going into AA. And the first thing I noticed was that treatment and AA were essentially the same thing.

I found AA fascinating. It's kind of like a cult, but it was also helpful to me. I couldn't get enough of these people's stories. Even though many shared a similar message, I found them intriguing, and I really got into it. I did the steps. I found a sponsor and, later, I sponsored people. Before long, I had my charges dismissed and had started to read about harm reduction. I thought, "Well, this treatment program isn't very good at what they do. I can do a better job." At this point, I was so excited about recovery, I wanted to make it my new career. I went to school. I had maybe eight months sober at this point, and I thought I could become a professional 12 Stepper. My first semester, I met this professor (yes, Dee-Dee Stout!) that was pissing me off. At the time, I still felt my life depended on AA, and she had the nerve to suggest that I consider some other ideas.

But I knew I was on the right path. It feels strange to say "destined," but it's hard to think of a better term because of how everything went down. I had always prided myself on being an open-minded person. I now think I was operating from a place of fear when it comes to 12 Step-based recovery. I may not have realized it, but I was ready to hear something new, even if I didn't exactly know *what* that was at the time. It was weird because I was gravitating towards other people who also seemed to be yearning for different ideas about substance use and treatment, and who were equally open minded.

By the end of that first semester, I had fully transitioned from 12 Stepper to a harm reductionist. I've benefited from it tremendously. I believe in its principles, how powerful *any* positive change can be. I don't think the two are mutually exclusive—12 Steps and harm reduction. I think that they can be used in conjunction with one another.

I continued going to occasional AA meetings, but by my second semester studying to be a drug counselor, I wasn't as interested in the 12 Step approach. I was still interested in studying the history of AA, and exploring many of its ideas—studying the culture and history of the program—but I was no longer interested in pursuing it as a recovery strategy. Like I said, I still find *aspects* of AA useful, and I have tried to carry the best part of its message, practices and principles forward, though it *has been* tricky. AA's program hinges on having had a spiritual awakening as the result of the steps. That's the message that you're supposed to carry, right? I did have a spiritual awakening, of sorts, and maybe *some* of that involved the steps, but I found so much more help *outside* the program in the harm reduction approach.

Starting with my second semester, I was really putting together my best version of whatever works. I got more involved in training, particulars like motivational interviewing, which I immersed myself in. I guess if I have a message, it's this: develop your own style. I've always used humor. I don't mind being called a smartass. I wasn't always an easy student, and teaching me was kind of hit or miss because my attitude and approach to life and learning was still a little flippant. I certainly don't think that I was prepared to work in my profession, at least not through my classroom education alone. I think that's probably the case for any professional: classroom education isn't enough. To do your job, you need practical application and further self-directed study.

I got my first internship a couple years into school. I won't say where, but it was appalling. And I *knew* it would be appalling. People warned me, but it was what was available at the time. Usually, at this school, you do two semesters of internship at the same institution; however, I found my way into another place for the second semester. I knew the right people! If I had not made that switch, I probably wouldn't have lasted a second semester without losing my mind.

Thankfully, it all worked out. I ended up spending the next ten years working at the Stonewall Project, which I considered to be a harm reduction dream job. It is the proud legacy of Dr. Michael Siever, who became my inspiration. In those days, the Stonewall Project was hardcore harm reduction. The people there were characters—the staff there were creative and fearless. There was an air of defiance, but in a healthy way. We were encouraged to be ourselves. And it worked because, in the end, we really cared about the work. We really cared about harm reduction.

I found my niche. I loved working there and grinded through the years. During those ten years, I seldom took time off. I became acquainted with good harm reduction people and was able to speak at a lot of conferences. I began writing and speaking more, spreading the word about harm reduction. Again, I found the right people to help with the right situations.

To summarize, that's how I came to harm reduction. I just kind of landed in it. Luckily, it made so much sense so quickly that I didn't have to unlearn very much. By the end of my first year of personal recovery—and I'm going to use the word recovery; I have no hesitation to use the term, which doesn't upset me (but when I define later on what that word means to me that caveat will make more sense).

Experiences, good and bad, will always have something to teach. This is probably where I lean most on the 12 Step world. There's a big emphasis on sharing your experience, disclosing your personal experiences in recovery. This concept did clash, slightly, with what I learned in harm reduction, which was, "Get over yourself, help the person with what *they're* dealing with— meet them where *they're* at in order to help them with what they're dealing with." Keep your inspiring stories of recovery to yourself rather than suggesting that what you did will necessarily work for this person. I'm here to do your thing. And that's just what my job requires of me: for me to get out of myself.

I don't need to have had your experience to be able to empathize with you. In fact, sometimes having the same experience makes it more difficult to empathize because I may project my experiences onto you. That can be dangerous. A bond forms, which may not be healthy, and eventually you'll discover, no matter how similar your situations, you are still two very different individuals. Self-disclosure will eventually break down when experiences diverge.

Back to recovery. For me, it's a broad term that refers to mental and physical health. It applies to trauma; it applies to substance use problems. Whatever ailment is troubling you is blocking you from living your life fully. Recovery means regaining that ability, or in some cases expanding aspects of your life for the first time. Kenneth Anderson of HAMS says recovery means, "I had a problem and now I no longer have that problem." That pretty much covers it for me.

When you see a psychiatrist, it's generally accepted that you don't go cold turkey off of a medication you've been prescribed for years. You go to a therapist. It's basic training that they don't tell you what to do. Instead, they were there to help lead, guide you to find your *own* answers and solutions. There're all these fundamental principles that are part of *any* good treatment. It all revolves around, "First, do no harm" and the autonomy of the patient. That's the governing precept of harm reduction: don't be an instrument of harm, and do not try to take away a person's autonomy. Like medicine in general, a provider must first commit to doing no harm. Telling people what to do, demanding immediate abstinence, practicing "tough love," and demonizing drugs and the people who use them, are all harmful.

Yet, that's controversial. Why? It's controversial in the 12 Step community because many of them still seem to think that until you hit rock bottom, you're never gonna get better; and that you can't even start working on improving your life until you've quit all drugs. That's the notion that a lot of people seem to have. Your life must get as miserable and wretched as possible before you can take any steps toward improving, which seems so counterintuitive to treatment for *any* condition. You wouldn't tell a cancer patient, "Sorry, we can't treat you until you hit Stage IV." No, you want to address the malady as soon as possible. A great deal of very meaningful work can happen while a person is ambivalent about substance use and change, and even still in the throes of chaotic drug use and its consequences. That's what harm reduction is: you engage with the person in the here and now. You love people unconditionally and help them with whatever they are motivated to work on.

You're not "bad" because you use drugs. I'm here to challenge you to harm yourself less. Michael Siever would frequently tell patients he does not care whether you use drugs, but he does care about whether you have a good life with or without drugs. That's how I view caring: you're challenging patients to see that they can do better, and you're helping them, however you can, to *do* better. And to do that right, you can't be judgmental or have an agenda. This is the message I got loud and clear from all of these discussions on harm reduction. With respect and autonomy, you can help others move toward a better place if they want to change. And if they don't want to change? That's fine, too. You still treat them with love and compassion, and perhaps the change they experience is being accepted while they continue to use drugs. "The curious paradox," wrote Carl Rogers, "is that when I accept myself just as I am, then I change."

Having participated in many harm reduction conferences and written, talked and thought a great deal about harm reduction philosophy, I have learned about the great people who came before me in this movement. Many of the most important changes involved breaking unjust laws and helping the people who need it by any means necessary. The movement is about people who use drugs. For me, maintaining that focus unites us, but in recent years I have noticed that many people in our ranks promote divisive identity politics rather than focus on reducing drug related harms.

I have been very disappointed in recent years to see people in harm reduction moving away from the fundamentals of the movement built over many decades of hard-fought activism on behalf of people who use drugs. It seems that many people now active in the harm reduction world are more interested in identity politics than trying to reduce drug related harms. At a recent conference, for example, I gave a talk on the importance of helping people not only reduce the harms but also increase the benefits of drug use. The title of the talk was "Just Say Yes to Drugs." During my talk, I casually referenced (mind you in a favorable light) that many hip-hop artists celebrate the positive effects of cannabis. A "wokester" in the crowd insisted that this comment was "racist," and that country music artists talk about drinking but I am singling out hip hop due to the prevalence of black artists. This person did not know me, and thus did not realize that I have been in love with hip hop since I was ten years old. This is just one of many cases of "woke" people trying to make harm reduction just another opportunity to shout down and cancel people because we have the nerve to talk about anything other than identity politics.

Let's get back to the basics of helping people who use drugs rather than allow harm reduction to become another casualty of the cancer of cancel culture.

Jeremy can be reached at jpharmreduction@gmail.com

ZACH RHOADS

had my own issues with drug use and an over reliance on drugs and alcohol throughout a good portion of my late teens and into adulthood. I did the whole AA experience. I listened to people tell me that I had some sort of malfunction or disease or faulty hardware, character defects. I think I *did* benefit from the social aspects of AA. AA was an opportunity to talk to people whom you can actually talk to about things like my drug use history and more. I don't know about others, but I can't open up in a lot of situations. AA gave me a place to go and share and meet others like me. I learned that I wasn't alone in what I was doing or what I was feeling.

On the other hand, I knew there was something different out there for me that was better. I knew I was more than my drug use. I really didn't want to be defined as "diseased"—I've done *good* things too. And when some of the guilt went away, I was able to be open minded, which allowed me to pull from a ton of resources on my road to recovery.

One of those resources that I soon found was the work by Stanton Peele. I had no idea at the time that he was seen as such an outlier in the recovery and treatment fields. His work really spoke to me. I emailed Stanton Peele to see if he'd be interested in doing a podcast with me and to my surprise his response was, "Sure!" That blew me away. Now we've done years of this podcast together including webinars, written a book together, and more. I still can't believe it sometimes.

Back in the beginning of my recovery journey, people would say that they admired my work or related to it. But then when I start talking to them, I couldn't understand why they were saying that because they didn't really agree with what I was saying. But when Stanton and I first connected, he kept engaging me, asking, "What do you think about this? What do you think about that? What do you think about human development? What do you think happens when a person does A, B, C, or D?" It was a terrific conversation. He kept in contact, which I thought was the coolest thing ever! He even asked if I'd be interested in writing a book with him. I wasn't sure what I had to contribute but was honored he'd ask. All this helped me move toward a more balanced life, one away from a diseased—or character-defect—label. It all added to my finding purpose in my life.

I came into harm reduction in an academic sense, not just in a personal one based on drug use. It was a natural fit. It made sense to me; no one had to twist my arm—I wasn't kicking and screaming. Because I've worked for many years in school systems with children who have various challenges, harm reduction was logical because that's how you work with children, especially those who have special needs of some kind. Harm reduction always made sense to me because a person in distress is going to use whatever tools they have at their disposal to help them cope. And so I could say, "You just shouldn't do that!" or "Shame on you!" but these kids have all heard that before and it's not helpful. I naturally tend to lean into what a person is experiencing, asking why they are doing the things they're doing, and this is especially true when it comes to children. I also always bet on them to outgrow their biggest challenge, whatever it is, as long as they have somebody to talk to, to coach them, or help them out. I try to be that for these kids I work with so there's always been a harm reduction element to my work.

I talked to a man named Tamla Summers, who wrote a book about honor culture called *In Defense of Honor*. I remember asking him, "How do you define 'honor?'" And he said that he couldn't—that it's a method, a way of living that involves a spectrum of what it is and how people operate. It's almost like the Observer Effect, where you can't pinpoint *one* thing because it's all moving around. I think the same thing about harm reduction.

A lot of different concepts are like that, encompassing a mentality and a way of life that embraces working with people who have some challenge in some area, or are engaging in certain behavior that's destructive to them. How do you best help? First, you need to understand why they're engaging in that behavior, or at least view them through a lens that sees them as human. With that respectful lens, you then help them discover resources that enable them to make positive steps in their lives, regardless of how they're behaving or whatever their lifestyles are like.

More specifically, I would like harm reduction to become more of a mentality and way of life. I would like it to evolve into itself. I came to harm reduction with a mindset that people *will* develop given the opportunity. We all grow, one way or another, so we need to meet people where *they* are, not where *we* are. People move at their own pace; they always have.

I hope harm reduction can move beyond the space of it being *just* about drugs and alcohol. I would like to see it move past any one subject and become more about how we treat human beings, in general. More respect. I do worry much like Carl Hart says in his book *Drug Use for Grownups* about the words "drugs" and "harm" becoming too associated with one another. I also wish people knew just how practical harm reduction is.

One high school I worked at had signs on the walls saying, "Please throw your paper towels away in the trash can when you're done," and of course people didn't do it. So they made more signs, like, "Please just do it," that kind of thing. Eventually, to solve the problem, custodians—not administrators—stepped in and solved the issue with one more trashcan and moving the trash cans closer to the paper towel dispenser. That's a practical solution to a problem. There's a practical level to harm reduction. You might not like what a person is doing, but if you're a realistic, honest person, you're going to acknowledge people will always use substances.

At a practical level, humans—like parabolas—are all over a map; you can't control it. I wish people would stop trying to control it. That's one thing. Then there's the ethical side. People really do develop. We need to recognize that in the recovery community. I think that we dehumanize people so often, we think of people doing their most destructive behavior, and that this will be who they are forever. Of course as a society, we must view some issues as intolerable. There are certain crimes that we can't abide because we don't want a crime-ridden society. I'm talking about hurting other human beings, offenses such as murder, etc. But even some death row inmates, and I've talked to a few, still find ways to provide—find ways to be useful in society—despite behind locked up. The point is most people *want* to grow.

When we work with people who engage in self-destructive behaviors, we have to search harder for the ethical approach. We still have to acknowledge that this person we're talking to is a human being, someone who can develop and probably *wants* to develop out of that behavior. I'm talking about doing *whatever it takes* to get people to acknowledge two things: 1) people don't have to be in this hole forever and 2) they might be if that's how we treat them.

Zach can be reached at zrhoadsconsulting@gmail.com

EDITH SPRINGER

Going back to the sixties when I was a drug addict, we would all sit around and talk about what we needed. It turns out that what we needed harm reduction. Years passed and I became a social worker. I went to work in drug treatment in a methadone program. Although I was doing well, my supervisors kept saying I was enabling and being too nice to my patients. I was having a hard time and I couldn't really understand the 12 Step model. I also couldn't understand the methadone model of having people come in every day. I just didn't understand that. This treatment wasn't nice to people but I was trying to accept and learn it. Then around the 1980s I went to work as a trainer at MDRI drug research because they needed someone who knew about AIDS. My friend Louie was a gay man who knew about AIDS and he brought me in to help me. We were at MDRI and my boss came to me one day and said that there was a guy from Liverpool and that he wanted to talk to my boss. My boss didn't have time, so I talked to this guy named Allan Parry and, oh yeah he blew me away! He was saying all of the things that I had been thinking and also what they were doing in terms of treatment. He was incredible! He made fun of me when he met me by saying, "Oh, you're in recovery. Where are your bandages?" He told me [a better solution) was to actually give people drugs. In Liverpool, people were doing this treatment and clients were getting better had families and jobs. Their treatment was working out really well. Allan Parry told me they were even giving out needles to teach people how to shoot up properly.

By the end of the conversation I was crying. After this, I took a trip to Liverpool and I saw everything that was going on there. I went to outreach with them. I went to the clinic where they gave out oranges and other drugs. Dr. Don Marks (at the clinic) looked at the methadone program and asked, "Why are we giving them only methadone and not heroin and cocaine?" People started to live normal lives and have jobs and bring their families together. Crime rates went down, so the police were in favor of it. It was like a dream. It was this wonderful thing and they called all of this harm reduction.

Then Margaret Thatcher came in and closed it all down. Before I left Parry's house, where I had been sleeping in Liverpool, I got on my knees and said, "I'm going to bring this to America if it's the last thing I do." And that's what I did. I came back to America and started trainings. I started a few programs in harm reduction. I trained three thousand people a year. I taught drug workers about harm reduction and it caught on. So I went back to Liverpool and then I went to Holland. I went to Sweden and all different countries to learn what they were doing in harm reduction. God, I went from town to town training people and I always stuck with harm reduction. And then we opened up programs in New York, and then other people opened programs in New York. We opened up a center in neighborhoods where people shot up drugs. We opened our tent and we gave out our services to them in tents. We did all sorts of services in that tent: counseling, HIV testing, helped people get off of drugs, and all kinds of things. That's how I really learned about harm reduction—from doing it.

What was different about us is that we didn't force harm reduction on people. We taught users to give up drugs slowly. They gave up drugs by harm reduction instead of what the 12 Step method was telling them to do. The 12 Step method was telling them that they couldn't work if they were using drugs. We were showing people that working helped to get people off of drugs because they have something to look forward to and to feel good about. *We showed them that they had a purpose.*

I read a book by the sociologist Erving Goffman. He said that the most destructive emotion is shame. And, the healthiest emotion is love. We tried to give people love and feel good about themselves. We didn't shame them about their drug use. Wow. That approach worked. A lot of people gave up drugs or reduced their drug use [because] they wanted to bring their families together. A lot of people didn't know about harm reduction but more people reduced or stopped using drugs with our method than the 12 Step method. They loved our programs and they felt *good* about our programs. We had a lot of programs in New York that were run by different people. We did a great job. The state health department gave us grants and that did a lot of good. The research showed that it was working.

To me, harm reduction is a method of helping people reduce harm in their lives in ways that work and that aren't emotional and judgmental but are scientifically based and actually work.

It's not just for drugs. People used it for weed (cannabis) control and other issues where they can't stop doing something that's harmful to them. It's a method that believes in any positive change. Slow change works better than fast, and it's filled with love.

It would be great to see all drug treatment programs use harm reduction methods and philosophies and it's great to see government funding now for these programs. I'd like to see drugs legalized or decriminalized. I'd like to see drug treatment programs actually maintain people on their drug of choice—like they did in Liverpool. That they put people on heroin maintenance and cocaine maintenance and then they find that it allowed them to live normal lives, stop committing crimes, get jobs, and produce positively to society. There's research to prove this. To see that happen, and stop stigmatizing users because stigma is a spoiled identity.

I wish that people would understand that harm reduction is not against abstinence. Abstinence is *part* of harm reduction. Harm reduction is not an evil thing. (Somebody called me the devil once for promoting it!) Harm reduction is not encouraging people to use drugs. It's helping people to get off of drugs. And if they continue to use, it's helping them to be safer in their practices so they don't get AIDS or other diseases. That's what I would like to see.

Edith can be reached through
deedeestoutconsulting@gmail.com

PART 4

FAMILIES & COUPLES

HARM REDUCTION & FAMILIES[1]

Family means no one gets left behind or forgotten.

...David Ogden Stiers

Treat people as if they are what they can be and you help them become who they're capable of being.

...Johann von Goethe

Hanging out with a friend, twenty-six-year-old Danny, a white, suburban male, took a pill. One pill. One pill that contained a highly concentrated, unregulated drug used to prolong a narcotic's effect. A few hours later he was dead. For Danny's mother, Louise, the loss has been immeasurable. Some days she can't shower. Others she can't get out of bed, the absence of her son leaving her "raw."

"It's been a nightmare," she says. "The cops said that they can't really do anything about it. There are so many homicides in Baltimore [where this happened]. They said unless there's an actual stabbing or gunshots ... wounds to the body ... [t]hey just don't have the manpower." Before adding, "I guess if you want to kill somebody, Baltimore City's the place to do it."

Danny, a young man who was just getting his life back together, liked to have fun, he'd still enjoy a drink or two, and this fateful night he'd thought he could keep the party going by popping a benzodiazepine. Unlike the anti-anxiety meds prescribed by a licensed physician or psychiatrist, Danny got his Xanax off the street. He split the pill with a friend, John. John lived. Danny did not.

This luck of the draw is called "The Chocolate Chip Effect." The term was coined for the efficient potency of bathtub fentanyl because of the way it can pool and isolate in minuscule but powerful spots. In this analogy, fentanyl is the chocolate chip in the cookie. Maybe you have a taste and get the chocolate chip. Maybe you don't. Maybe you live. Maybe you die.

Danny's mom Louise, an emergency room RN and fervent advocate of harm reduction, acknowledges that some people are going to keep using drugs. [Harm reduction] says, "[L]et's reduce the chance of killing yourself until you can make better choices."

And she has tried to use her son's death to help others, starting with his memorial and funeral service, where Louise handed out Narcan, an opiate overdose revival agent, as well as fentanyl test strips.

"There were probably two hundred kids at Danny's funeral," she says with bittersweet pride.

John, the friend who survived the night Danny did not, joined in helping hand out the Narcan and strips. By the end of the service, all but a few of each were gone. Louise acknowledges she is not the first parent to suffer such a loss, nor is she the first to hope her child's death will be the last.

"I want to stop other parents from having to go through this," she says. "He took a pill," Louise says. "He wasn't out robbing houses to get high."

"My son mattered," she says. "And he will always matter to me, and if I can keep this from happening to some other mother [I will]. Because nobody deserves this."

***

Kendra opened the door to find her son dead from an overdose. She had long before decided that in order to keep Jon alive, she would not only buy his drugs but have him use in the family home, in the downstairs bathroom, always with the door open, so she could hear if he fell or cried out that something was wrong. This was the hardest decision she had ever made but it was the only way she could sleep at night since his return home from his 5th rehab in less than two years for his drug use. She was determined that her only child would not die in the streets so what other choice did she have now?

As I write this new section of the second edition of *Coming* to *Harm Reduction* in the summer of 2024, we've seen some 110,000 deaths from drugs in the US, mainly from mixing various drugs, which has always been the deadliest way of using drugs especially illicit ones. We are in a crisis of overdoses. However, to be honest, we still have nearly 500,000 deaths a year from smoking- related illnesses. And the Alcohol-Related Disease Impact application estimates that each year there are more than 178,000 attributable <u>to excessive alcohol use</u>, making alcohol one of the leading preventable causes of death in the United States, behind tobacco, poor diet and physical inactivity, and illegal drugs.[4,5] Yet we hear very little about tobacco and alcohol. Why? Because they are legal (or licit) drugs and so we as a culture have decided to accept these drugs even though more harm is caused by them than most illicit drug use. Drug use here in the US is as complicated as the two opening real-life stories demonstrate. And every family must find their own way to endure their loved one's addiction, and possible recovery, however they each choose to define that.

In the second edition, I knew I wanted to have a chapter devoted to families who 1) have used some non-traditional ways to help their loved ones and 2) want/wanted a way to help their loved ones without using "tough love" or worse the now too often deadly "let-them-hit-bottom" concept. Here I've also added several stories from families—as well as some case examples from my work with families using Harm Reduction Psychotherapy or HRT—of those who have used harm reduction or "non-traditional strategies" to help their loved ones with an addiction. These same harm reduction strategies have allowed many families to begin the healing process sooner and make healthy changes for themselves regardless of the outcome of their loved one's attempts at changing their relationship to a substance. At the end of this section, you'll find a few basic Harm Reduction Psychotherapy (HRT) concepts that many of the families I work with have found useful when designing their *own* change journeys into something often called *recovery*. While nothing works for everyone and certainly not for all families, my hope is to give readers and families an idea of how anyone might begin to have deeper conversations with themselves and others about what I call *The 3 "L's" of Holistic HRT for Families:* **love, limits,** and doing what you can **live** with.

Taking harm reduction principles and strategies and applying them to working with families might seem to be a new concept and, in many ways, it is a novel way to think about harm reduction and harm reduction therapy. Though looking closely at some early experiences in my own work with families in drug treatment, I think harm reduction has always been a part of my work and others', too, though not as pronounced as it could be or is now. But we'll get back to this a bit later. For now, let's travel back to the start of my work with families to see how I and the field got to where we are today.

A Very Brief History of Family Work in Addiction Treatment:

I've worked with families since the early days of my career in the late 1980's. Developing and running family programs in social model treatment programs was something I came to enjoy and did many times over the course of 15 years or so. Of course, I mistakenly thought *I* was teaching participants something about their role in their loved one's addiction along with the basic concepts on addiction and recovery, when really, they were teaching *me*, because what I really needed to learn was how to listen to *them*. I'm grateful I am finally learning how.

In the beginning...

It was in 1951, 16 years after the start of AA, that Lois Wilson, AA co-founder Bill Wilson's wife, is believed to have first discussed publicly that wives (remember, no one considered couples to be anything other than heterosexual back then and men were the main "alcoholics") also needed support while their problematically drinking husbands sought a new relationship with alcohol—abstinence—in AA.

Family programs in addiction treatment were available in nearly all drug treatment in the late 1980's and early 1990's. This was also the heyday of the 12 Step, this-is-your-brain-on-drugs, abstinence-only Minnesota medical disease model of drug treatment, and when we first saw the terms co-dependency, adult children of alcoholics (ACOA), and other (mainly white) middle-class, heterosexual, nuclear family, socially constructed ideas of how an otherwise healthy family structure would become dysfunctional at the hands of a family member who was using substances, sometimes problematically. Out of this time came experts such as Melody Beattie, Sharon Wegscheider-Cruse, and Claudia Black, all teaching families and the majority culture that substances were the cause of nearly all our family's problems and destruction, and that the only solution was to confront the "addict" about their substance use, require them to enter formal, typically residential treatment, or lose access to the family's love and support. And so, in the midst of this volcano, the worst concept of them all, "tough love," was born (more on that later).

In residential treatment, the identified patient (IP) was typically not allowed access to their family members unless the family was participating in Family Group. Families were seen as problematic to the work the treatment agency and staff were doing with the patient (this also included outside therapists and doctors). Even phone calls were often limited to once weekly and were brief, on purpose. In those days, the role of treatment was to cut off the IP from all external influences that were believed to be hugely problematic to their lives and certainly to their recovery. However, once the family had completed the Family Program, connected with Al-Anon and had met with the client and therapist, they were considered "in recovery" themselves. Typically, a conjoint (a meeting of the IP, their family, and the Primary Therapist) was scheduled just prior to discharge where the therapist would facilitate a meeting to encourage family members to be clear on the severe consequences suggested if the IP returned to drug use. The IP was also to begin the process of making amends to their families for the destruction their addiction had caused. I just realized today how much we were furthering the shame we knew the patient had under the mistaken belief that this shame would keep them from returning to drug use and allow the family to heal.

Through her lens of one attachment theory, our hospital's Family Therapist, Ashe Maranthe, taught me the importance of relationships especially in families where someone had an addiction; how patients viewed their family members and how family members viewed their loved one using drugs. This was the early 1990's and we had a free yearlong 1.5 hour-long Family Group as part of the continuing care (we purposefully didn't call it *aftercare* like many other programs as we felt treatment was a beginning not an end) we offered for both patients and family members. For an added fee, our hospital rehab also offered a week-long Family Program Intensive run by another lifelong mentor of mine, the late Mickey Marsh, PhD, MFCC who held a doctorate in Human Sexuality. Family members would stay at a local hotel and come to a location off campus to meet with others also challenged by an addiction in the family. Here they would learn about the disease of addiction, codependency, family roles, support groups (AlAnon or NarAnon were the only ones available in those days and AlAnon was seen as superior) and learn that they were *also* going to need to make changes if their family member's treatment was going to be successful.

Mickey Marsh used to say she had a black belt in AlAnon. Her last husband, the late Dr. Earle Marsh, had been the Chair of the OB/GYN department at UCSF and one of the first doctors to teach other doctors and medical students about addiction. He also still has the distinction of being the only story in the Big Book of AA that includes drug use (as he tells it, he was addicted to methamphetamines as well as alcohol). Plus, his original sponsor in AA had been its co-founder, Bill Wilson. Doc Earle, as he was called, was also part of the rotating experts we had at the hospital, often speaking to patients about sex (he was hugely sex positive, mainly to raise endorphins in those recovering brains but also just for joy) as well as nutrition, meditation/spirituality, and of course, AA. The Drs. Marsh were beloved by all and I'm confident they both would be proponents of holistic harm reduction psychotherapy today.

OK, so now that we've discussed a bit about the theories used to create family programs back in the 1980's, let's move to what we should be doing with families today. Sadly, the biggest change I've seen in rehab is the exclusion of family programs or the severe shrinking of them at least. It seems ridiculous to think that we could take one member of a system out of that system just to return them to the same system and not expect negative results for all. But this is all too often what happens. Gratefully there are folks out there who focus on working with families in addiction and especially who do this from a harm reduction perspective. Let's discuss what I mean by that now.

The Intersection of HR/HRT and Family/Couples Work

If harm reduction psychotherapy (HRT) is a method of client-centered counseling or therapy that has multiple parts to it, then *HRT with Families & Couples* will be just as complex. It's also very creative and flexible, offering clinicians working with families and addiction treatment to do so individually as no two families are ever alike in their resources, needs, or goals. This is what traditional family work in addiction treatment too often forgets.

In all harm reduction work, we value and center the voice of the individual. Therefore, in Family & Couples HRT, a large part of our job is to value and center the voice of the family. This isn't easy as many times family members have differing goals or needs. But this strategy can lead to a conversation about *negotiation* as well as learning to view the family/couple as another entity. I prefer to use the term "negotiation" to "compromise" as too many people hear *compromise* and think, "Oh boy, what I am going to have to give up!" The word *negotiation*, though, says each person will get *some* of what they want/need. It's also a more positive perspective and that's what we want: less focus on problems and more focus on solutions and what's going right.

When I first started learning about family dynamics in addiction treatment, we used the term "co-addicts" to describe family members. The idea behind using this term was to show that the person addicted as well as the family member(s) *all* begin to behave in less healthy ways, a parallel process of maladaptive coping if you will. Reading about codependency again for this new section, I was struck by how the "diagnosis" of codependency (remember, there is no actual diagnosis as codependency is not found in any DSM) is based on someone *else's* interpretation of your behavior. This is one of the problems I have with the term. For example, as one writer and advocate of the term states, one characteristic of codependent behavior is *one person handling the finances because "they're better at it,"* *rather than encouraging the other person to learn those skills* *themselves.* If my partner is genuinely better at finances and I'm better at fixing the car, why is that a problem versus a division of labor? And further, a problem that needs a diagnostic label? Alternatively, what if we see this division of labor as each member of a system (a couple in this case) doing what they're good at, playing to their strengths? Of course, each partner should know some basic things about the finances (such as the institution where the finances are kept, where the checkbook and bills are kept, or what platforms are being used to receive and pay for things); ditto fixing the car. But each partnership or other type of family needs to decide for *themselves* what division of labor works best for them.

Of course, this is the problem with all labels: they are stiff, very black and white, and frankly unlikely to be of much use beyond some general conversation or theoretical musings (and insurance payments!). And yet we, especially here in the States, consistently insist on using them, harm be damned. Let's take this example from Patt Denning, PhD, coauthor of *Practicing Harm Reduction Psychotherapy*, now in its second edition. She states,

Maria was a married 27-year-old woman who came to the community mental health clinic where Patt was working. Maria said she was seeking family therapy to help with some family troubles. Her husband of a decade was working very long hours and to relax he would come home and drink excessively every night. This behavior was helping him unwind but also meant he couldn't help with their 3 children or help Maria with other chores. She was also becoming increasingly uncomfortable about calling into the office for her husband, making excuses for his tardiness or absences. To Patt, Maria's problems mainly seemed to stem from her husband's drinking. Since Patt's training led her to view Maria's behaviors as "classic codependency," she told Maria that she needed to stop making excuses for her husband's drinking as both were now hurting their family. Patt also gave Maria a referral to a standard alcohol and other drugs treatment facility for her husband to hopefully receive treatment and for Maria to learn more about her "codependent" behaviors. Patt states that she was pleased with her assessment of the situation and felt she had done a "good job" referring Maria since while Patt was trained in marriage and family counseling but certainly wasn't an expert on alcohol and drug use. However, Patt says after a conversation with the treatment facility, she was a little uncomfortable as it seemed they were only focused on this perception of how Maria's behaviors were contributing to her husband's alcoholism and not viewing the family system as a whole, as Patt's clinical training taught her to do. But they were the experts.

About 6 months later, Patt met with Maria again after she called asking for therapy. Maria said she was grateful for Patt's help and that the treatment center had "saved my life." However, the family was in trouble in other ways now. Patt's own words continue here:

*With the encouragement of her alcohol counselor and the group members, she had stopped protecting her husband. When she stopped calling his employer to make excuses for his absences, he was fired. Despite advice and confrontations from the counselor and the group about how she should divorce her husband, she found that she just could not leave him. After he lost his job, the family of 5 was now dependent on welfare. The husband's "recovery" (abstinence from alcohol) was intermittent, and Maria was overwhelmed. Evaluation showed Maria to be anxious and dysphoric, with insomnia, hopelessness, difficulty concentrating, and irritability with the children. She expressed both fear and resignation regarding her husband's alcoholism and her continued ability to help him and her children. I was alarmed and distressed. **What had I done? What help did I give her?** (emphasis mine; p4 – 5)*

Denning goes on to say that she learned a lot that day—and that she would never again mistake someone's coping behaviors for codependency even when they may be problematic. As Jane-Peller would say, "don't confuse preferences with problems." If we're not going to use the old ways of viewing all family systems impacted by addiction as problematic, how should we view them? One way to improve our view of these systems immediately is to give compassion and validation to all family for doing their best in typically awful circumstances. And yes, that includes the family member using problematically!

When we begin to see that addiction is often a response to a traumatic event or extreme situation, we can begin to comprehend how anyone, even one of you, might be tempted to turn to substances to cope. Remember: it's not the substance but rather what it does for someone that leads to the addiction. Drugs are merely doing what we designed them to do: relieve some distressed state or help us to feel more elated, relaxed—better than we feel right now.

Are there some "bits and pieces" of HRT I might use with families that are also in keeping with some of the traditional Family Therapy concepts I learned so long ago? Absolutely.

I often start by asking about the values of each member of the family, including the member using substances. One thing I like to do with many of the families I work with is to ask each member to separately complete the Personal Value Cards Sort. However, rather than follow the instructions provided, I ask them to come up with their Top 10 most important values from the list of some 120 values (or they may make up their own of course) and bring them in some form to the next family session. In conversation with the entire family, if possible, we then go one value at a time to discuss *how they know this is of value to them*. Sometimes I ask them if I were watching their behavior, what would tell me that this value is important to them? For example, the value of humor is important to me. You would know that by listening to me talk as I nearly always manage to get some laughter into whatever I'm doing, even a session!

Another thing I'd like to know more about is what the family knows about addiction or why people use drugs—so I ask! I often include some education about the Stages of Changes and the theory called "Drug, Set, Setting," if they allow. I might also discuss the many ways people change (and yes there are many. I have a shelf full of books telling me this) and usually something about how all harm reduction includes abstinence (it just doesn't demand it). By the way, this last part *always* surprises everyone.

Lastly, I'd like to know something about the state of communication in their family, especially with their family member using drugs. Often there's no direct communication between the family and their loved one using substances. Sometimes there's one person in the family that the member using drugs will speak to or perhaps a trusted family friend, but they aren't speaking to their direct family members. Typically, by the time families get to me, they've a) already been told about the traditional ways to get their family member "clean and sober," b) they've spent a financial fortune (one family I worked with had spent $250k by the time they got to me), and lastly c) they're exhausted and frightened and angry and overwhelmed and don't really want to hear what I want *them* to do; they only want to hear how to get their loved one off drugs. And I understand.

I also want to let them get to know *me* as I get to know them so some personal disclosure on my part often helps build trust—which I rightly need to earn, not expect, from any client. Finally I need to answer every question, honestly and direct-ly. That means I'm often saying, "I don't know," which can be frustrating. But my job isn't to tell families and couples what to do or give direct advice (with great exception)—after all this is their family not mine—but rather my job is to listen deeply to them: their dreams, their desires, their fears, what they've tried already, what has & hasn't worked and where they each are now in this process. Mainly, I need to know how much they can honestly invest in this work right now. Everyone I know who works in harm reduction with families tries their best to be aware of resources of all kinds and accommodate as best we can. At the very least we can be honest about that, and sometimes we're the first professionals who have been.

The very last thing I say to most families is that while I can't *ever* guarantee the outcome of our work on their family member's drug use, I can almost guarantee that they, the other family members, will feel better about what they are doing, or not do-ing. When families are a bit less stressed out, more ideas of what they can do and won't do, and an actual roadmap to wherever *they* choose to go, is also more imaginable. At the conclusion of our work, I would like each family and each family member to know how to communicate better with each other, to have some basic knowledge about how change happens, under-stand why we all use drugs, and develop a more realistic, balanced view of what they can control and what they can't. Most of all I want them to have hope. And I am a proud enabler of it!

I also want families to know that their family structure is unique and therefore their roadmap to recovery or changes will also be unique. Our first goal in Family HRT is to keep the lines of communication open with their family member using substances, or to repair that communication if at all possible. If that's not possible, we can work on the communication between the rest of the family members, which is often strained too. Parents often can't agree on how to handle their child's drug use while they are still living at home; couples argue about the amount their partner should drink at a party, and more. And lastly, while exiting your family member is always an option, I always ask families to please make it the *last* option not the first. Most importantly, if you make a threat to exit your family member or something else, you'd better be prepared to follow through or else future limits will not be taken seriously.

I want to end this chapter with an excerpt from the interview by a new pal, author Chris Grosso, with Dr. Gabor Mate, in Chris' book *Dead Set on Living*. I often use this excerpt in the classroom when teaching the next generation of therapists and counselors as a great example of "out of the box thinking" especially in their work with families and couples in addiction treatment. It is by far the best example I know of a new way for families and others with loved ones problematically using substances to conceive addiction. And it always leaves me breathless and in tears. Perhaps it will touch you as deeply too.

Chris met with the eminent physician and addiction expert, Dr.

Gabor Mate. They were speaking about families and Chris said he felt his family had done everything they could to help him, but Dr. Mate disagreed with that assessment. Instead, Mate said that of course Chris' family had done everything they knew to do and that nothing worked; he wasn't arguing with Chris about that. However, he said that didn't mean there was literally *nothing* else they could have tried. Perhaps they could have said something like this:

We recognize that your addiction is not your primary problem ... you're in a lot of pain. And that pain is not yours alone. [It] has been carried in our family for generations... You're just the one who's soothing it with that behavior... Thank you for showing [how much pain there is in our family] to us... We're going to ... [heal] ourselves. We invite you to be there if you feel like it. And if you're not ready ... then just do what you need to do right now.

Chris goes on to say that Dr. Mate was certainly not saying that his parents were to blame for Chris' addiction. He just wanted to show Chris—and all of us—that there are indeed other options, other ways of viewing addiction. However, each family is also free and should have limits or rules around whether they can maintain some contact with their loved one in addiction. The other part of this conversation that is crucial is that if you're going to have your loved one who's using substances in your life, then you must accept them right where they are and stop trying to change them. What we can't do is to remain a part of their lives and nag or threaten to try to change them. If we do that, we're only saying to our loved ones that they are not enough the way they are, that in order for us to truly love them, *they* must change and be who *we* want them to be.

To me, one of the most important things Dr. Mate states in this excerpt is to recommend that families not try to change the family member using substances. So, what can we do instead? We can focus on improving communication or find reasons through conversation that our family member might want to make a change in their drug use or offer to assist them *however* they *want* when they are ready to make any positive change. In the meantime, I hope families will hear that there's much they can do for *themselves* which just might have a positive effect on all their family members, those using drugs and those not. What isn't OK is to focus solely on the family member using substances because the change the family may want might never happen. I believe it would be awful if this kept you from having *any* relationship with that "problem" family member because it will hurt you as well as the rest of the family...and it may mean that you won't be around when your family member decides to examine and possibly change their relationship to substances. This is why HHRT/HRT Family and Couples work in addiction is so very important. After all, we can hardly ask our loved ones using substances to work on themselves if we're not willing to do the same ourselves.

Endnotes

1. The term family here will be used for ease of reading and includes all groups of concerned people: couples, friends, traditional/non-traditional families and more.

2. Dr. Earle Marsh had studied with Alfred Kinsey, participating in some of his early research on human sexuality.

3. "Demystifying Codependency" by S.M. Stray in Medium, 8.12.2019 (accessed 8.14.2024).

4. Denning, P. & Little, J. (2011) Practicing Harm Reduction Psychotherapy, 2nd ed. The Guilford Press. NY, NY.

5. These are available for free at https://www.motivationalinterviewing.org/sites/default/files/valuescardsort_0.pdf. There are also a variety of ones available for sale at Amazon and other retailers.

6. Dead Set on Living, by Chris Grosso (2018) Gallery Books, NY/NY. p25-6

THE 3 WORST WORDS IN ADDICTION TREATMENT: CODEPENDENCY, ENABLING, & TOUGH LOVE

Feelings of worth can flourish only in an atmosphere where individual differences are appreciated, mistakes are tolerated, communication is open, and rules are flexible - the kind of atmosphere that is found in a nurturing family.

...Virginia Satir

Like the well-known fear trio of the past, *"lions, tigers and bears, oh my!"* in family addiction work today there are still some basic cliches for any of us who love or work with people who use drugs. These well-worn words and phrases are repeated often to families who are vulnerable, scared, and often desperate for help.

1. You are codependent & must get help to stop aiding your loved one using drugs

2. You're enabling your loved one to continue to use drugs

3. You must let your loved one "hit bottom" or they'll never going to learn and change

"Why should they stop using drugs when you're making it so easy to continue?" people will say. All of these comments may even sound sensible on the surface, but they lack an understanding of motivation and what drives basic human behavior and change. They also assume we have more power over our loved ones using substances than we really do. What we know from decades of studying human behavior is that motivation is encouraged more by loving-kindness than with anger and threats. One example of a way to look at this phenomenon is to examine the rates of recidivism from prison. A U.S. Department of Justice analysis of recidivism rates in 24 states concluded that 82 percent of individuals released from state prisons were rearrested at least once during the 10 years following release. Within one year of release, 43 percent of formerly incarcerated people were rearrested. If prison, which is one of the worst "bottoms" in life most can imagine, were positively associated with motivation and change, then we'd have little recidivism, right? Clearly that is not the case. Why do we continue to culturally insist all too often on using a stick (punishment) and not a carrot (reward) when it comes to people who use substances?

Codependency

[Codependency] can mean sooo many things...

– Melody Beattie, YT interview, 2023.

We can see evidence of this interesting idiom all throughout addiction treatment—with clients, their families, and others. *Drug use is bad so it must be punished; families and others must stop enabling this terrible behavior, but they struggle to do so because they're codependent so "tough love" is the only answer for all of these groups.*(emphasis mine) While these three concepts intersect, let's take them one at a time. We'll focus on the concept of *codependency* first.

Codependency is about the relationship you have with yourself. It's a set of characteristics and patterns of behavior we develop to help us cope, typically from a childhood that revolved around (but is not limited to) addiction, emotional instability and trauma, and physical or mental illness.

The concept of codependency can be traced back to the German psychiatrist, Dr. Karen Horney, born in 1885, who coined the phrase "tyranny of the shoulds," a symptom that inflicts many codependents, especially women. She saw it as the self-critical persona that develops from the anxiety formed by neurosis and a yearning to become our true selves. Self-criticism and low self-worth are two of the many characteristics of codependency. Certainly two that I possessed and still often struggle with. (Carol Weis, PsychCentral article; 9.13.2017)

1986 was the year the first edition of Melody Beattie's ground-breaking book, *Codependent No More*, was published which went on to sell more than four million copies and stay on the *NYTimes* Best Seller List for 115 weeks. A drug counselor,

Ms. Beattie, who holds no degrees or special training (except for a high school diploma), became *the* expert in this thing called "codependency" as a result. Though Beattie didn't invent the term, it was her work that led to the concept exploding into our culture. Soon there were treatment centers offering help for "codependents," those family members of "addicts" who were clearly responsible for much of the "addict's" drug use, so they said. This was quite confusing to many since Al-Anon states, "You didn't cause it, you can't control it, and you can't cure it." So, which is it? Are we family members responsible for our kids/partners use of drugs or not? Either way the message was clear from all corners: the only thing families could do was, "Let go, let them hit bottom, and detach." Really? Perhaps those were the only choices in 1950 when AlAnon began, but are they *still* the ONLY choices in 2024? This is my first problem with the term(s).

A second problem I have with the term codependency is who gets to decide who's codependent? As Jane Peller, LCSW, former Professor of Social Work at Northeastern University in Illinois and a mentor of mine, once said to me, "Don't confuse *preferences* with *problems*." Who am I to say that someone's *preference* to have their child at home while detoxing is wrong? Or perhaps they pay for a room for their loved one chaotically using substances. Is that wrong? In many cultures, being dependent is seen as both powerful and necessary for survival. The concept of codependency can be seen as an affront to those cultures (and I've seen many rehabs push this concept onto vulnerable families who would never have otherwise made the decision to remove their loved one from the family as a "stick" or punishment for using drugs). In many Western cultures, especially here in the US, we tend to dislike the idea of dependency; we value *independence* as the highest goal even if this is an impossible task. This thinking has certainly contaminated our concept of addiction treatment, including working with families as well. Of course, the truth is none of us are "self-made." All of us depend on someone, or someones, for help. Many mental health experts now worry about the lack of connection we have with each other, even going so far as to calling it an "epidemic of loneliness." Yet, the primary "treatment" for families with a loved one who is using substances is to tell them to disconnect from that loved one. How is this sensible, let alone good science or medicine? Are we just perpetuating the hate that most addicts feel for themselves with this "treatment?" How can this concept possibly lead to mental health and wellness?

The third major issue I take with this seminal book is that Ms. Beattie claims there are 11 pages of symptoms or characteristics of codependency. With that number, everyone in the world could fall under this label or diagnosis! This is also part of the reason that codependency has never been accepted as a diagnosis by the APA. It's simply too broad. Recently, in response to the term "codependency" there has been a movement toward the term "prodependency." According to Psychology Today staff writers:

Some experts are advising that we move beyond codependency and adopt alternative ways of managing a relationship with someone who has an addiction or mental illness, including prodependence. This strategy allows caregivers to love unconditionally and pursue an emotional connection while simultaneously developing and maintaining healthy boundaries. Someone in a prodependent relationship will offer help when a loved one needs it but not do tasks that the person should (or could) manage for themselves. Emphasis mine.

As I was recently listening to Ms. Beattie in a 2024 interview (touting her new edition of *Codependent No More*, now focusing on anxiety and trauma as part of the constellation of causes), I heard only binaries from her: black and white thinking. Good family therapy or counseling of any type should be the opposite of that. We clinicians need to be open to all possible options or how will we help families discover what path is right for them? Since all families are unique, there is absolutely no one who can tell you what to do that will be guaranteed to be helpful to your loved one using drugs. Let me say that again, bluntly: if any professional tells you that the *only* way your loved one will stop using drugs is for you to do "XYZ," run, don't walk, out of that office immediately. Just because we're well educated and experienced does not mean we have a crystal ball to tell the future. We should be able to say what we suggest based on your particular family dynamics but, first, we should ask questions like these: What sounds right to you to do right now? What do you think would work with your loved one? What has helped and/or made things worse in the past?

So, instead of giving folks a label or "diagnosis" based on an outrageously large collection of characteristics or symptoms, how about we help folks to improve their communication skills? And perhaps we could also help folks focus more on discovering and creating limits with people that they love? Why do we have to choose between loving ourselves and loving or doing for others, especially family and friends? These binaries are in my opinion what gets us in trouble, every time. My experience is that sometimes those in counseling or support groups for codependency wind up becoming quite self-centered, rarely offering to flex a "boundary" of theirs for a friend/family's need. How is this loving and kind?

Enabling

I'm a proud enabler of HOPE.

– Dee-Dee Stout, 2023

The next word on my "hit list" of the 3 worst words in drug treatment is "enabling." I believe it's one of the places we can most easily begin to reinvent or reframe some of our language. Typically, I hear this word used constantly to mean something negative, that somehow I'm "allowing" a harmful or risky behavior to continue, as if I or anyone has such powers. But the word doesn't have to mean a negative. I'm a professor. I sure hope I've enabled hundreds if not thousands of students to learn more about various topics over the 35 years I've been teaching. If not, well, we won't even go down that road. *Enabling* means to help, make able to, allow, permit, or to provide the means or opportunity. So yes, I can negatively enable someone as well as positively enable them. In drug treatment we often tell families and others that they are "enabling" their loved one to continue to use drugs by paying their bills, giving them a home to stay in, calling into work when they're hungover. And yes, all of these *could* be negatively enabling. But they can also be positive: Mom has found that a large wine helps to relax after work most nights leaving her daughter to pay the bills so the lights stay on and the mortgage gets paid. Or how about the parents who decide to keep their son at home as much as possible (he's had a few stints at the ED after overdosing) so if another trip is needed, the parents can drive him. The last time he was admitted to ED, the doctors called him a "drug seeker" and left him to suffer for hours alone. Or the how about the parents who learned to dole out cannabis to their son because it helps him better manage his symptoms of anxiety than pharmaceuticals. It could also mean that they are enabling their child, partner or other family member to stay alive, literally.

One of the things these scenarios all have in common—besides the fact that they're actual situations from clients of mine—is that each family came to their own decisions after trial and error and sometimes conversations with harm reduction therapy professionals like me. Also, in each of these cases, families—that's *all* members including the person using substances—decided on some "bumpers" or guidelines for everyone. In the case of the mom and daughter, they decided that mom would do some of the bills on school nights and what didn't get paid would be left to the daughter on Sunday night. The parents decided that thinking about their son living on the streets was so stressful, that they would rather have their son live at home. And there were some bumpers about how that would work: who would do the cleaning, take out the trash, how they would make decisions that affected all living in the house, and more, just as you might with any other living situation with multiple people.

There are many, many ways to make life better for our loved ones engaging in risky behaviors. One thing I often ask couples is, "What risky behaviors are acceptable to you?" The first time I asked that to a girlfriend of a client whom she worried would die from drug use, she didn't quite understand the question. So I gave some examples: "You know, swimming in the ocean; riding a motorcycle with a helmet (or without); hang-gliding; driving on the freeway in the Bay Area. All risky behaviors. Which of those are acceptable?" We have all been battered by the idea that using drugs, especially illicit ones, is a death sentence. And yes, sometimes it is. However, basically it's one risky behavior and life has risks—and we can learn how to be safer about our substance use. I want couples and families of all kinds to learn how to have these difficult conversations about risky behaviors and values in life. After all, if we're willing to shut the door on a loved one due to their behavior, don't we owe it to them—and to us—to have a non-dramatic, low-key, fact-based conversation with them first? I think so. And this leads me to my *"3 Brief Takeaways for Better Communication"*:

1. Have conversations when you're calm. There's enough drama in our lives. Soap operas belong on TV not in your home.

2. Use concise *chunklets* rather than have "The Talk." I often suggest folks set their phone timers for 5 – 10 minutes only, especially at first. And no bringing up past "bad behaviors."

3. Absolutely acknowledge what's gone well! Anthony Kiedis, frontman of the Red Hot Chili Peppers, once said, "Mental health isn't a 24/7 thing." He's right, especially when we're talking about addiction. No one engages in any behavior 24/7. It's not possible. So be sure to "catch in" your loved one for doing what you've asked or hoped far more than you "catch them out" for doing things wrong. John and Julie Gottman, of the famed Gottman Institute in Washington state, have studied and worked with thousands of couples and they say that we should complement our loved one at least *5 times for every negative thing we say to them*. Yeah, this is going to take some practice!

Tough Love

The American National Institutes of Health *says that "get tough treatments do not work and there is some evidence that they may make the problem worse."*

When we expect immediate changes and refuse to be with the person during the process, we undermine the very goal we seek to accomplish.

— Tony Trimingham **I**
Founder, Family Drug Support, AUS

Instead of defining Tough Love, let's end with a discussion of what love is. Love is a singular word in American English but can have a few similar meanings: Oxford Languages suggests that love is "a deep affection, fondness, warmth" for another; Merriam-Webster says it is "strong constant affection for and dedication to another." In the Bible, 1 Corinthians 13 is often cited as how the apostle Paul saw Christ's teachings, encouraging his followers to see love in this way: *Love is patient, love is kind. It does not envy, it does not boast, it is not proud. It does not dishonor others, it is not self-seeking, it is not easily angered, it keeps no record of wrongs. Love does not delight in evil but rejoices with the truth. It always protects, always trusts, always hopes, always perseveres. Love never fails.*

When I asked AI to define love, here's what it said: *Love is the act of putting others before oneself.* All these definitions would seem to be opposite of what the concepts of codependency, enabling, and tough love are based on. To me, and again when working with families and couples, I ask *them* how they see

love. It is frankly completely unimportant and perhaps dangerous for me to consider or push on them how *I* might define
love. My job—the job of all of us in the helping professions—is
to help others (families) navigate their own journey, to examine what *they* want and don't want, not replicate some unattainable cultural ideal of what healthy families do, seemingly
based mainly on old television shows. Why? Because my interpretation of a healthy family may not be the same as yours, nor
should it be. This is the main problem I have with t*ough love*. It
says all "addicts" are "liars, thieves and cheats" and all families
"are codependent enablers." Would we speak this way to families coping with other illnesses? I certainly hope not.

Now I can also appreciate the dilemma of the family. They're
often suffering and stuck; they don't know what else to do because whatever they've tried so far has left them angry, sad,
confused, and their loved one hurt and alone often. Let's remember why I used drugs for 20 years: because I was in pain.
I despised myself for being "an addict" because I thought it
meant I was a failure. Actually, what my drug use did was help
me cope with some things in life that I had no tools to cope
with. Sadly, the tough love that I experienced left me using
more drugs more often as I became more and more isolated
from my family that I had always depended on. And the more
pain I was in, the more I was left needing to numb out. This is a
typical experience for many of us long-time chaotic drug users.

Mainly I hate tough love because it's anything but love—not for
families and not for those family members using drugs. In fact,
I think we need to get honest about tough love: it's anger, rage,
at those who have disappointed us, or it's vengeance for the

hurt and pain caused by those using drugs. And that's really why our culture has been mostly OK with tough love for generations: tough love says, "This is what those dirty drug users deserve for breaking the rules of society." Meanwhile, we drug users are desperately trying to find ways to continue to numb the pain we're in. Dr. Gabor Mate likes to say that "hurt people *hurt* people" and he's so right.

In harm reduction psychotherapy work, and especially in *HRT for Families & Couples*, we really want to do everything we can to remove or reduce thresholds to our loved ones thinking about a possible change in their relationship to a drug. What do we mean by thresholds? Envision your front door. You probably have a threshold that you walk over to get into your house which helps keep the door from leaking air among other things. Now imagine if you will that the threshold has suddenly grown so much that you have to get help to get boosted over it. If you had to do this every day for the rest of your life, what decisions or options might you try? Might you even consider giving up? This is what it can be like for your loved one to get into treatment or access some type of help. Harm reduction says, "Come as you are" and we who practice HRT say, "and leave as who you want to be!" A colleague of mine from Maine, Stephen Andrews, likes to say, "Meet people where they dream." What a concept, huh? When was the last time your loved one was asked about their dreams? Maybe they've even stopped dreaming because life seems so hopeless. I've been there, just like so many millions of others. And someone didn't let me just stay there. Instead, they accepted me, right where I was in my active addiction, treated me like a human being, and slowly, inch by inch, I began to change my relationship to drugs, and mainly to myself. I started to really believe that another life was possible, something I pushed against for 20 years. Patt Denning and Jeannie Little said it well in their book *Over the Influence* (2011):

In a society that values independence over dependency needs, children's needs for attachment are frustrated, sometimes resulting in an attachment to things that are not human—like drugs (p80).

Bottom line: Families are individuals and as such are unique. What's right for one is wrong for another, which is why it's impossible to give advice that holds for all families. But we can talk about a few basics, which start with encouraging everyone to treat each other with respect and compassion—nd keep in mind that you're all doing the best you can at any given moment, even if it's not helpful right now. So, as we move into some general guidelines for "OK so *what can we do?*" let's remember what I call the *"3 L's of HRT for Families & Couples*: **limits, love**, and doing what you can **live** with. Finally, start working on yourselves. You can call it recovery or wellness or whatever you like but the absolute best way to help your loved one using drugs is to start making your own changes. Modeling healthy behaviors is a terrific way to influence your loved one's behavior. It takes time but, in the meantime, you'll start to feel better and that might also positively influence your partner or child. Remember what flight attendants always tell us: *Put your own oxygen mask on before helping others*. It's also a good motto for families and others to use when loving someone who problematically uses drugs. Whatever you decide to do with your family, I wish you well. And please remember, *do whatever you can live with and make peace with it*. Good luck!

Resources

You'll find information on books, workbooks, websites, and professionals that families and I have found useful over the past decade posted on my website at <u>deedeestoutconsulting.com</u> under *Resources*. Then look for the *HR-friendly Resources for Families & Couples* section. Many also have podcasts attached which you'll easily find on their individual websites.

Endnotes

1. Nov 27, 2023.

2. https://al-anon.org/blog/al-anons-three-cs/

3. https://harmonydust.com/wp-content/uploads/2019/03/Characteristics-of-Codependent-People.pdf

4. https://www.psychologytoday.com/us/basics/codependency#:~:text=There%20is%20no%20scientific%20research,Statistical%20Manual%20of%20Mental%20Disorders.

5. Ibid.

6. 1 Corinthians 13: 4-8 NIV.

BRENDA ZANE

didn't really know harm reduction was a thing, an actual thing, until the last few years, when I started working with so many families. I discovered that too many parents had been told "100% abstinence is the only option" by every professional they saw. Now I'm talking to drug users who are adolescents and young adults between 13 and maybe their early 20s and what we're seeing is that a lot of times that goal of complete abstinence just doesn't work. In fact, it often gets in the way of making any progress with these young adults. You tell a 16-year-old that they are never, ever going to touch a substance ever again—well, that doesn't go over so well. So, I knew harm reduction in theory, the concept of harm reduction, but I didn't know the actual phrase or name for this "less than 100% abstinence" concept. I just didn't have any sort of really good harm reduction education or information. It's been a journey.

This means too that I may define harm reduction differently than others here. I look at it as finding ways to adapt my behavior that makes life tolerable or enjoyable in a way that also does less damage to myself or to a person's overall well-being.

And that could be, as I was thinking about it, related to food or exercise. You know, we have so many choices with food—what we put in our bodies, how much we move our bodies, and more. That's how I look at harm reduction. It's really when there's an option to do something that's safer or that will have less of a negative impact on me or someone else and I choose those actions as a way of keeping myself healthier, safer.

I would really like to see harm reduction being better represented in addiction work with adolescents, because that's where so much of *my* work is done. Right now, what I see happening is that parents who start to embrace harm reduction are often then told they're enabling their kids. And it gets really confusing for them. I would love to see parents and families get the message. I would love to see more understanding, ways for parents to embrace harm reduction with a teenager *and* hold boundaries—because that's the other part where parents often tend to fail. There's not a source of education for parents around this—how to work with harm reduction and not feel like they're enabling their kids.

What *I've* seen is how working with such harm-reducing concepts such as Community Reinforcement and Family Training (CRAFT) and motivational interviewing (MI) often will open conversations—and the opportunity for conversations—so much better than the old methods, which really weren't about conversations anyway. By using MI and CRAFT, we can then often move that young person closer towards being safer or even potentially being abstinent. And frankly we would love for the adolescent brain to be abstinent—it clearly isn't ideal for the health of the developing adolescent brain to use substances. But if not abstinence, having kids be *safer* when they use substances would be an improvement. The challenge I see is that these conversations aren't able to happen if families are in a power struggle. This is especially true when there's a battle over 100% abstinence.

It would be great if parents could learn how to set boundaries, and I think harm reduction conversations could help here. For instance, how do I say, "Okay, seventeen-year-old, if you're gonna smoke weed, I can't stop you. I don't agree with it or like it but I sure appreciate you telling me." And then we start to discuss where or how I set some boundaries around that use. Let's say I don't want it in my house, or I don't want it in my garage. How do we do both harm reduction and set boundaries with our young folks? I think that's what's missing for families. We need a way to believe in harm reduction and practice harm reduction, or allow our children to practice harm reduction, while keeping us all healthy and safer, and not feel like we're doing the wrong thing. That's really what I'd like from harm reduction—and I think it's getting there.

Brenda can be reached at http://hopestreamcommunity.org

CATHY TAUGHINBAUGH

My path to harm reduction came through learning more about the community reinforcement approach (CRA) and CRAFT as the parent of a child who had a difficult relationship to substances. That's also how I came to the work I do now with families. I learned at the very beginning of my journey with my child that an abstinence-only approach is what we do in this culture, what we're told is the only way forward—your child is either sober and in recovery, or they're not. It's black and white. There's no other option. I didn't know that there were other paths to recovery or positive change until much later. When I learned about CRAFT, and now Invitation to Change (ITC), I began to understand that there are indeed more options. I've also learned that we need to empower people, we need to respect a person's ability to choose their change process. I've learned that viewing our loved ones this way—as independent and needing to choose how and what to change for themselves—can really help with *our* stress as well as our loved ones'. You know when someone is struggling with their substance use, the strategy of being told what to do is not very helpful. Instead, we need to help them bring their motivation and desires out of themselves, out of ourselves too. This was how I learned about harm reduction. Unfortunately, this was all after my daughter went through her addiction. Gratefully she is now in a much better place. Now I can step back and look at all the approaches. CRAFT and ITC make a lot more sense than what I was told when my child was in trouble. I really wish I had known then what I now know, which is why these days I work with families who are struggling with their child's substance use. And I get to share with them these other, more effective methods.

I have also come to define for myself what harm reduction means to me over the years. I've taken many different people's opinions on harm reduction and worked toward coming up with something that makes sense for me. So, I see harm reduction as a non-judgmental, compassionate approach for people who are seeking help. It's really about any issue too, not just about substance use because the goal is to reduce the harm that comes with substance use or any behavior. Harm reduction meets people where they are. It offers options with less risk and those could include abstinence, moderation, or continued use, if that person isn't ready to make more changes. But in my opinion, I think harm reduction moves people forward. It respects people and gives them the power. I think it's empowering to give people the chance to make their own decisions about what kind of change they want to have in their lives.

Harm reduction means meeting people where they are. It promotes the idea of reducing drug or alcohol use to safer levels, which I think is important. And I think the key to harm reduction is not turning our backs on the people we love, especially those who are not ready to change. We don't want our loved ones to come into the office of somebody—a therapist or treatment provider—and, if they're not quite ready to give up the substance, hear, "Well, I can't help you. Come back when you're ready to change." You know, there's a lot of growth that can happen in that time between formal treatment and ambivalence when we simply support any positive change our loved one can (and will) make right now.

I wish harm reduction strategies and philosophies were taught in more treatment programs. I'm still seeing parents being told their child just needs "to surrender" to the treatment program. I also hear these parents being told they need to stop voicing their opinions and just follow the directions that treatment providers give. That is so wrong. I would like these programs to see families as part of the team, and I'd love for this kind of teamwork to become an accepted practice.

Lastly, I think treatment professionals should use harm reduction as an option—one that's always available. And that addiction counselors should be trained in all treatment modalities, including harm reduction. There are a number of counselors who are in recovery, but they've gone through the abstinence-only approach, and that's great for them but it's so important that they have the ability to talk about and offer these other options. We can do harm reduction *and* other options. Let's talk about how we can all move forward in the best way that makes sense, to families and their loved ones. I believe our outcomes would be better and people would be more willing to get help [if providers were more open-minded]. I also think we would have more families intact.

That's on the provider end. I'd also like families to know about harm reduction. It's a missed opportunity when we don't individualize treatment, which is what harm reduction is all about. Families need to understand that harm reduction is moving somebody forward in a positive direction, and when people are offered options, it means more people are willing to get help. If someone feels like, "Okay, I want to get help. But I'm afraid they're going to make me do things I don't want to do right now," that fear comes up and gets in the way of them getting that help. And it's terrifying to try to make these kinds of changes we're asking of our loved ones sometimes. But if people knew that they would be able to move forward in a slower pace—small steps—then they might be more willing to try. Bottom line: families need to know that harm reduction saves lives.

Finally, I've realized that harm reduction applies to everybody, but I don't think we talk about it that way for parents and family members. I think parents need to look at harm reduction—what *they* are doing—how the isolation, the yelling, and more is damaging *their* health because dealing with a child with an addiction can be *years* of stress. We all need to think about what we can do around harm reduction for parents and other family members. Parents can minimize the harm that's coming by using harm-reduction strategies. These could free them and other family members as well as their child from much of the pain that can be generated by an addiction in the family. And what a great help that would be for everyone affected.

Cathy can be reached at http://cathytaughinbaugh.com

CHERYL & MORGAN (alias)

Cheryl: Between us, we have eighteen years of drug and alcohol experience. Sometimes chaotically, sometimes not, sometimes a tiny bit sober, sometimes not. Unfortunately for Morgan, I put her into a therapeutic boarding school that further traumatized her. The rehabs I sent her to didn't help either. But that's all I knew how to do. This is the definition of insanity. I knew there had to be something else out there. I started to Google, which is how I found my way to medication, like methadone, which Morgan had agreed to try. I used to think of that as harm reduction, but I don't anymore. It's more than (how we define) medications.

Morgan: I always knew what harm reduction was. I never could relate to it. I thought I was doing everything I could. But really? I just thought I was cooler than everybody. I thought that I could escape death.

I definitely would not have been able to get sober if it wasn't for my son. And even that, there were still times where I chose drugs over him. To this day, I choose [destructive] behaviors. It took a long time to understand this. I didn't gain a conscience

395

overnight. It was more like I slowly started becoming aware what I was doing to myself.

My dad sent me a video. I was super high in a store, going back and forth, spinning, my son with tears streaming down his face. That was the first time that I got up and dropped everything [to get better]. I know if I don't do something different I'm going to lose him. But I can't stop using, so what can I do?

My fiancé is a wonderful example because he's sober. He's been clean and sober for ten years. He doesn't know the day he stopped using drugs, stopped drinking. He stopped drinking slowly. He prayed to whatever God you believe in—the Universe, whatever you call it. He got out of the *self* and in that game where consciousness [promotes] spiritual growth. Eventually all these character defects and the problematic behavioral thinking slipped away, one by one. That's what's happening to me. It's been a crazy spiritual awakening. I always knew I was addicted. I always knew I had an addictive personality. But like my maternal instinct not kicking in (at first), I thought, OK, this is not good, because my son's gonna grow up without a mom.

The biggest thing [in getting better] is being honest with myself, being honest with others. In doing that, I become more aware of everything else around me. I become aware of my insecurities and why I do this to myself. It's learned behavior to love the unworthiness of my childhood trauma. And it's not working anymore. It hasn't for a long time. Harm reduction has let me hold up a mirror to myself. And I don't like the person looking back. I want to do better. Drugs and alcohol kept me alive. For a while. Because I would have committed suicide without them. I would have tried to check out a different way. But enough is enough. I want to be like my mom.

Cheryl: People don't understand. My own family doesn't ask questions anymore. They don't understand. That's why I started my own group. I had nowhere to turn where I was not being shamed. For loving Morgan—the good, the bad, the ugly and everything in between. I'm not perfect. I get down sometimes. I'll say to Morgan, "Okay, I'm retreating for a couple days. I need to check out of the chaos. I'll be back. Don't worry. If you really need me, you know where I am. I'll just cocoon for a couple days, and then I rise again."

Morgan: I need my mommy. I don't want to do the things that make her cocoon anymore. I want her in my life. I want her to love me through all this.

Cheryl: I don't have the skill in terms of drug policy, but I read every morning for two hours and post [to my group online]. I have friends who've lost their kids to drugs—it's not just about Morgan. It's hard. Sometimes I need a day to regroup and rise again. These are difficult stories to listen to—my kid is out in a park, and … I had my husband buy her drugs, because that was the only way she was going to come back with him to the hotel room. We need to have her safe, give her drugs, and make sure that she keeps the door open to go to drugstore, to get Narcan. We let her use drugs all the way home. And all the way through methadone until she got stabilized. She was willing to try something different. So we did too.

When I started sharing stories like this in the group, people were attacking me, telling me that I was going to kill her because, yes, sometimes I would give my daughter money. Sometimes I didn't. Sometimes my heart said, You know, if I don't give her the money to get drugs, she's gonna get the drugs anyway. She'll prostitute herself to get the drugs. I don't want her to sell her body or her things. People would say, "You're killing her! What if she uses it, and she overdoses and dies? That's going to be on you!" It was just awful, awful, awful. So I decided I'd start my own damn group and get away from people like that. And I did.

Morgan: Harm reduction showed me what stability looked like, because I have no routine. I had no routine. Think about how upset babies get when they don't have routine. Now imagine how upset adults will get when they've never had one.

Cheryl: So you have [a culture of] secrets, which might end in death. Morgan's just now getting totally honest with us, and we've been at this for eighteen years. [Reestablishing] trust doesn't happen overnight. I wish I knew then what I know now. Because I could have shaved off years. I could have helped her more.

Morgan: But here we are, and she's still as you can tell, walking, talking, mothering, doing the next best thing—the next right thing—baby steps.

We talk about this a lot, celebrating those little things, how any positive change is progress. Hydrating more? Eating better? This is harm reduction. If you're taking methamphetamines, try to monitor your last use so that you can get some sleep. [My mom's] so sweet about it too. She knows how much shame I have, the guilt, how I beat myself up. That's what we do: we stay in our shame. If there's nobody helping us, nobody's there to cheer us on, then what? I don't have bigger cheerleaders than my dad, my brothers, my fiancé, my son, unknowingly. But my mom's my number one cheerleader.

Cheryl: I'm wrapped up in the drug and alcohol aspects of harm reduction. But harm reduction can be applied to much more. I was tickled when they started slinging harm reduction around talking about COVID-19. This word is now being used. It's the same principles: it's ways to reduce damage. Harm reduction [also impacts] decriminalization and incarceration issues. At the heart of the War on Drugs, there's a lot of racism. You're talking to a couple of white girls here, but that's how politicians and opponents (of harm reduction) view people that use drugs and alcohol. It's systemic.

Yes, I apply harm reduction to my life, personally. Even if it's something simple like stepping out and bubbling up. I have to remind myself not to allow stress to overtake me. Which is what will happen if I don't sleep or eat enough, if I don't meditate and get my soul in the right place. Everything goes out the window. Compassion goes out the window. Anger and fear come around. I'm not the best version of myself. I reduce harm by taking care of myself so that I can be a better person and a better mother to a person that's struggling.

Morgan: For me, there really isn't one definition. I think it definitely involves meeting people where they're at. You're not trying to force people into treatment or rehab or to get better. You're trying to acknowledge the use drug use or the alcoholism, and work with the user to make it safer and keep someone alive. In the end, I think harm reduction is its own category. On a global scale, harm reduction is more than drugs and alcohol; you can apply it to all areas of your life you want to work on.

Cheryl: A user isn't powerless—parents are not powerless. We *are* powerless over [a lot of] our children's behavior, but we can educate ourselves. We can read and listen to experts in the field of mental health and addiction. We can align ourselves with the best people studying this. We can listen to evidence-based reporting and research to cut through all the media crap.

Morgan: My fiancé always says to me, "Give yourself a chance." Give yourself a chance. You can't rush your healing. There's also a song by Trevor Hall I love: "You Can't Rush Your Healing." It's an unbelievably beautiful song. I recommend it to everybody. It's about how the darkness teaches you and you can't rush the healing part because everything works the way it's supposed to.

If people had more information, or there was one person who could tell them that they're going to make it or that they can amount to something, no matter how small the achievement, no matter how small the change—that they're worthy of having a good life—maybe they can hang on till things get better. You don't have to hurt yourself or feel shame—harm reduction serves *every*body. Harm reduction is about healing. It says we are always going to be fighting the good fight, if we don't give up on each other. That's how I feel. If it wasn't for my family not giving up on me, my partner telling me that I'm safe, that I'm loved—and I've heard every day—I wouldn't feel safe and I wouldn't feel loved, and change wouldn't be possible.

DOUG & JANE (alias)

Doug: Jane and I had gotten into a relationship. We had been very close friends before. Once things transitioned from friendship to relationship, I think it became more important to be healthier. When we first got together, we struggled with my drug use. Jane had seen me as a friend. We'd party, try new substances. As a boyfriend, I was seen differently.

Jane: Because as his friend, I was further removed. I knew that he used drugs—he'd kind of joked about addiction. It wasn't something that personally or intimately impacted me until we were dating.

Doug: When she pointed out this relationship had changed, I did not want to admit it. I didn't want to do any work. Which is a human trait (I hope!)—it's definitely one of my traits. I had done Cocaine Anonymous and Alcoholics Anonymous, which was court ordered, I had done therapy, and we talked about my addiction with a more traditional therapist who essentially said that it was abstinence or nothing. I didn't try that until I got arrested on multiple drug possession charges. Though 12 Step wasn't mandated this time, it looked better if I was in the program. In order to fight my case and try to stay out of prison, I did everything I was supposed to. I did randomized drug testing. I had bouts of sobriety for randomized drug testing. I also learned what they test for. I remember being at a party with a friend and saying to him, "I'm not having *any* fun—I'm *so* sober." He's like, "What are you talking about? Your eyes are like dinner plates!" And I was like, "Yeah. Mushrooms and LSD, but I can't do any cocaine or smoke weed!" I had struggled with that. I'd had a complicated relationship with drugs, and I continued my use despite negative effects to my life.

I struggled a lot with abstinence. I felt controlled. I felt a *lack* of control. I wanted something that had less shame and guilt, because I was crumbling under the shame and the guilt of [failing to be abstinent] so long. There were all these voices in society telling me I was wrong—that I was a bad person. There's judgment around drug use. I had heard about harm reduction. I Googled the term. I looked through a couple of the results. Nice websites. Okay, I said to myself, this looks cool. I didn't know anything about harm reduction, not formally. Jane and I went to the office of a renowned harm reductionist. I didn't do that seeking harm reduction, as much as I wanted my partner to see me taking some steps towards [recovery].

I really appreciate abstinence as *part* of harm reduction. It's great—if you can pull it off. Harm reduction helps remove the stigma and allows you to carve your own path, which is different than abstinence. It took me a long time to find harm reduction. My health was suffering. I ended up with a perforated septum. I wasn't sleeping. I already had some issues like a deviated septum. When I was in my twenties, I couldn't jog or run. Total muscle failure. Serious stuff. I normalized it. Under abstinence, I'd do okay and then suffer these big bursts of use, which were very harmful. I carried so much shame and guilt. When I got harm reduction, I was, like, "Okay. I might not be the worst person in the world for doing this." In the beginning, just finding a way to hate myself less was a blessing. Addressing *all* your problems doesn't happen overnight.

Jane: This was a difficult journey for me, getting to know Doug's addiction, intimately. I had to be careful not to trigger myself. The situation brought out all of my abandonment issues. I was at the point where I was up all night long with anxiety. Is he using? Is he okay? You drive yourself crazy with that thinking. I found myself trying to control and manage his addiction, which of course isn't my role or responsibility. Eventually, we got to a place where I was like, we need someone who is specializes in this, because what we're doing is not working. How I'm handling it is not working. We were struggling to manage the problem. We needed professional help. At the time, I didn't know what harm reduction was, and I definitely struggled to grasp the concept. I didn't actively seek it out. It's more something that came as a result of understanding what harm reduction was, being open to it, being honest with our journey.

Doug: There's a lot of the professionals out there who will outright reject harm reduction. They'll say, This is not good. This is enabling. This is, you know, toxic, essentially. I think we struggled with the concept at first because there were all these other voices, or couples therapists who I think meant well, but who actually hurt our relationship. My own (personal) therapist, who I'd been seeing for several years, was still hammering home abstinence, abstinence, abstinence.

Addiction is weird, [in that] it's socially acceptable to shame others. Harm reduction offers different pathways to recovery. You can have a little binge now and then. You can be abstinent. Both are part of harm reduction. Whereas abstinence-only is just, you know, you go to the meeting, you read the book, you repeat the thing, you wake up, you go to the meeting. And if you should relapse? You lose your tokens. There's this walk of shame. It's like, "Oh, I used to have this many years sober, but I used last night so none of that matters."

Jane: The way that I understand [harm reduction]—and I'm still learning about it—it's about meeting people where they're at. What's best for that individual person? Or what does *that* person need? And to Doug's point, it took me a long time to accept abstinence is not always the answer, that it's not so black and white. You can't force something on [a drug user] that they're not ready for.

Doug: I have a lot of vices. I try not to shy away from admitting that. And I have many complicated relationships with many substances. To me harm reduction asks a simple question: Can I do something healthier tomorrow than I did today? It's a lot of two steps forward, one step back. Progress is not necessarily linear. I think the "progress not perfection" crowd doesn't always understand the "progress" part. The "perfection" aspect (i.e., abstinence) is still part of the equation. If you just slip up even once, they'll bring it up. I remember a guy with twenty years having a drink, and at the next meeting he stood up and said, "I'm not going to give this up just for one stupid day." And I thought it was weird, but it was really relatable to me. He beat something and was abstinent for twenty years. He had made a victory every day for twenty years. And to give that up, I mean, what is that? Almost twenty-thousand days? No, it's more.

There is still this weird struggle with harm reduction. Because it's chaotic, it allows for backsliding—progress is not linear in harm reduction. Sometimes it's hard to define the end goal, right? I would like to see it being *more* empowering, like, "Hey, I'm taking charge of my relationships, and I'm not perfect. And it's not always going to be great. But I'm trying!" There is this weird patriarchal element, which in our society claims it's all or nothing—if you're not first, you're last. Abstinence fits that mindset; harm reduction doesn't. We have strong social forces at play that undermine harm reduction. Because it's cooler to sit around and say, "Oh, I drank so much!" than it is to say, "Hey, guys, last night I drank a little less than I normally do." That's great. Did you still feel fucked up? Sure, and it was healthier. High five. That doesn't happen.

Jane: I remember taking DARE classes as a child. They instilled this idea that all drugs are bad drugs. As I was starting to use, exploring my own journey, I had to remove the shame.

Doug: At first there is this weird, toxic cycle. It's fun. You're like, Oh, I'm so bad. I'm such a bad boy. Look at me being so bad. Like, I'm actually so bad. And then you're like, Oh, I'm such a piece of shit. And it's gone from having fun by playing in the gray area and doing something naughty, to feeling like you're a terrible son and a bad husband. I was always a good student. I was well behaved. [Reckless drug use] was how I acted out. "This is me being a punk!" [What I learned from] DARE helped fuel that. Later on there'd be people wearing real DARE T-shirts and doing a lot of drugs. That propaganda will actually incite kids to do more of it.

The problem with being in a relationship is that you're dragging your partner through the suffering. That's the part where drug use and relationships gets so complicated. The first few times with Jane, we'd use and have all this fun, and then we start going to bed and I just want to do a shame spiral. She's like, "What's going on? We had a good time!" That shame spiral is such a big part of addiction, and it's so dangerous for relationships.

Jane: For me, understanding [harm reduction] meant accepting [recovery] is not a linear path—there is no *one* path. And you can change the path at any time. Abstinence didn't work for Doug. And so he sought out harm reduction. As his partner, I have to ask where I fit in. To get better, you need resources and understanding for the people, partners, family, or friends who are going through this journey with the person that they love and care about. How can someone better support their partner?

Doug: Couples need to talk about it, open and honestly. Where at first, I thought [helping me] was an act of control. Now I ask, "Is she doing this because she actually cares about me?" This is an act of love, right? It took me a long time to be like, Oh, she worries about it *because* she loves me. She wants to spend more time with me to make sure that I'm healthy. But if I don't look at it from a risk tolerance gap perspective, then it's like, "Why is this person being so crazy?" When I look at how I use today, the amount that I use is significantly lower, and the way that I use causes a lot less self-hatred. I don't know if those metrics [accurately] measure my journey but they *are* positives. With abstinence, it wasn't allowed. I wasn't allowed to ask, "Hey, why am I using? Yeah, why do I feel like I need to erase myself?" With harm reduction, one of the things that changes is there's no one that says, "Oh, you're bad, don't do this." Instead, you ask why am I doing this? Can I do it in a slightly different way? I feel like it actually opens up more room. At least for me it did. This stuff is so personal. It opened up more room to examine my own happiness or ask, "What am I learning from this experience?" "What are my fears?" It's helped me mature as a person.

What I like about harm reduction is how it mirrors relationships. Every day you get to work, every day is different. You kind of have to adapt and learn to communicate with yourself, learn to communicate with your partner. The big tool is being able to untie these little knots—these little trauma knots that tighten as we grow up. It's hard to say, "Hey, I used a little less!" Or, "Hey, I'm actually struggling or today, I didn't do so well, and I drank more than I wanted to." That takes vulnerability.

LINDA (alias)

In March 1984, I went into treatment to get sober. At that point, recovery, for me, was all about the 12 Steps. There were no other options. And back then, there was a very hard line drawn about what constituted sobriety. For instance, you couldn't be on any medication. Like many alcoholics, I drank to address underlying issues. There were times when doctors suggested that I take antidepressants. The official AA party line was always, "Oh, no, that would threaten your sobriety." I didn't listen to my doctors, didn't take their educated, medical recommendations because I was so fearful of what AA would think; I was worried they'd judge me. I was able to stop drinking without medication. I also made it much harder on myself by not addressing a chemical imbalance. This extra work was just that: extra work. And needless. It's changed today, thankfully. There is a difference between taking medications prescribed by a doctor and self-medicating. This is a vital distinction, and where I think harm reduction comes in.

I met my partner Derek shortly afterwards, while we were both students at the University of Santa Cruz. We'd been in a small group together working on a project. One day he asked me out. At the time I had one year of sobriety. Derek had three.

Derek was recovering from heroin addiction. My drug of choice was alcohol. Derek's three years seemed like a lot more sober time. And it is—in terms of time. You often hear in the rooms "a drug is a drug." That is true. But there *is* a difference between heroin and alcohol, ranging from societal acceptance—not only does society tolerate alcohol use more, it openly encourages it! Heroin binds to receptors differently, which presents its own unique challenge.

After Derek and I were married, we jumped in the treatment industry professionally; we were both trained for it. The idea was to use our past addictions to help others.

Derek got a management job in Contra Costa County. Then we started a clinic of our own, which we operated for twenty years. Now that we were "experts" in the field, we stopped going to meetings. It didn't seem like a big deal. We'd conquered our respective addictions, were helping others, and so what was the point? That was the problem: yes, we were helping others. This didn't mean we could—or should—stop working on ourselves.

And all it took was one day to have it all come undone.

Derek was in Berkeley, on his way to get a massage. He saw someone sitting there at the BART station, a guy who looked like he might know where to get some heroin. I guess that's how it goes, you know?

Derek overdosed that first use. He came to, several hours later. He was okay. But I didn't catch it. Derek was the last person in the world I'd worry about. Our clients and patients? Sure.

But not Derek. He was a pillar in the recovery community, from our own clinic, to helping at outside ones like Haight-Ashbury (which he continues to do). First, of course, he had to address his relapse, and as his partner, I was affected too.

Addicts, whether in active addiction *or* recovery, are always going to be flirting with that line of codependency. And even though it was just Derek who had relapsed, it wasn't just him impacted. I saw the personality changes. I didn't address it in a healthy way. We, his family and I, started to see it. His daughter started to see it. And these interpersonal relationships began to turn abusive. Maybe not *physically* abusive. But abuse takes all forms, and active addiction changes how people interact, whether they are using or abstaining. When you are involved with an addict, you can't help but become part of that story.

Derek was a tough guy. He didn't want to admit he'd slipped. He immediately went into that tough guy mode, which is a defense mechanism. We undermine the severity of our problem.

Addressing Derek's addiction meant operating in both worlds—helping others in recovery while we—and I say "we" because I was every bit in it too—fought for sobriety. I might not have been drinking. But I was, for lack of a better word, enabling. I mean, it was just so hard for me. I'd see the tracks on Derek's arms, and him fading, and he's say, "I have to go to the store. I gotta get ... something." I knew he was lying. I could see the pain he was going through. I loved him. I gave him money, so he could go on his way. And now I'm hiding the syringes I'd accidentally find.

Addiction is more than just the drugs. Pretty soon, I'm just as paranoid as he is! I'm locking our bedroom door, calling his brother, scared because I don't know what was going to happen. Or I'm on the phone, talking to a friend, and Derek picks up another line to eavesdrop, worried I'm having an affair. We'd gone from this stability to complete uncertainty.

Like I mentioned, we ran a clinic. I'm the director of the treatment facility. I think our employees knew before I did. Even though I knew Derek was using, I couldn't *see* what that meant. I was able to compartmentalize. We were the experts. *They* were the addicts. Derek's relapse wasn't the same as theirs. I know how crazy that sounds. That's what addiction can do. Employees started to come to me, voicing their concerns, but I couldn't hear them. I heard the words of course. But I couldn't come to terms with the problem. I didn't *want* to face it.

Finally, it just got too bad. It came to a point where one of the staff called me and we had a long talk, and my eyes were finally opened. It was time to address the elephant! We staged an intervention, and Derek agreed to go into treatment. Derek was a crazy man by this point. This was a rough-and-tumble facility, and Derek was coming up against some gangster types, and it was tense. Derek wanted to leave. I tried to be strong. I said, "No, I'm not going to pick you up." He called a taxi and came home. So it just kept going. But this was a start. The path to recovery isn't always a straight, fast line. It's two steps forward, and three steps sideways sometimes. Even though *this* attempt wasn't successful for him, there were still those moments where I'd catch his eyes and see he wanted to get better. He'd had *twenty-five* years of years of sobriety at that point before he relapsed. The foundation *was* there. It was just crumbling.

Everything came to a head when Derek got arrested. Police

planted a baseball-sized amount of PCP in his car. And as horrible as that was? In a weird kind of way, that was the godsend. We got Derek representation, and we had what the police planted retested, which revealed one inert substance. This in turn highlighted what the authorities had done, which ended up in everything getting thrown out. But it was a wake-up call. I think this incident showed Derek he couldn't let others have such a sway over his life and fate. He'd come really close to going to prison for a long time, and regardless of the misconduct by police, I think Derek recognized he'd put himself in that situation, giving them that power.

After he dodged that bullet, Derek called a friend, a colleague, and he started going to a methadone clinic. He went out of the county, because he didn't want anyone to know. Some people, like that first group I attended back in 1984, wouldn't see the positive impact of the methadone. To them, Derek would be seen as substituting one drug for another. Maybe so. But methadone was a bridge to recovery. This is what harm reduction is all about. He stopped scoring off the streets, got back to his work, and by mitigating the damage, slowly but surely, he got his life back.

Derek and I started attending a 7 a.m. meeting. Even then, he was still what they call "chipping," using here and there. But he was using less. The methadone and the programs started to work better, which meant he was cutting back.

It wasn't easy. In fact, it was often the opposite, knowing Derek was doing so well most days, but then still chipping, nickel and diming—it was driving me crazy. I wanted him to be fixed *right now*. I realized this meant I also had to change. Recovery is a never-ending process, and you can't let perfection stand in the way of progress.

It was baby steps. I remember this one night. We were living there in Port Costa, and we were both exhausted. We were up in the mountains, just walking. And then we both collapsed in the middle of the woods and started crying with each other. The burden. The journey. We knew it had to change.

Derek didn't stop trying to get better. He and I went to couple's counseling for a while. I have *my* own issues, which included suicide attempts. I think these thoughts of suicide were just like, craving a drink. It's part of my makeup. I'm used to it, the whole crazy ball addiction encapsulated. I had mentioned this suicidal ideation in one of the counseling sessions, and both Derek and the therapist about fell out of their chair! To me, it was no big deal. You don't know how you or your thoughts appear to others. This is a long about way of saying, you can't hold onto it all yourself. You have to let go.

Derek and I go to meetings every day. He now has almost twelve years of recovery under his belt now. We continue to work with people every day, helping them, and I think we are better equipped, as strange as that may sound, *because* of Derek's relapse. The experience afforded us an added insight and empathy to help us help others.

It's that inability to decide. Fear of making a decision. There's a couple other women, whom I sponsor, and they come and go. But I'm always there when they want the help. This is harm reduction: more better days than bad ones, until you put some serious recovery time in the rearview mirror, and the ground under your feet becomes steadier with each step you take.

There is another component that I need to address, which involves personal therapy. I am the survivor of sexual assaults

414

and other personal violations. This of course contributed to my drinking in the first place. I've been in a lot of therapy over the years. Meetings help. I also use a more holistic approach, which includes concepts EMDR (Eye Movement Desensitization and Reprocessing), which is a form of psychotherapy to address repressed memories. There is also something call "Hanna somatics," which is a neuromuscular education technique that employs both verbal and hands-on instruction.

For me, I've found all three of these—meetings, EMDR, Hanna somatics are like the ABCs of how I can be in this world. I'll also admit to seeking the help of a shaman! And it worked!

This might not sound like a big deal to you, but I grew up in a *very* Christian household.

I was with my sister a couple years ago. We went to go on these horse ride things, and she asked me if I believed in Jesus Christ—as a savior. I made it very clear. I said, "I'm glad that works for *you*. But I work with what helps *my* recovery."

So much of recovery is just that: understanding, accepting, and respecting what is right for the *individual*. One-size-fits-all works for hats; it doesn't work for recovery. To me, that is another aspect of that harm reduction: peace and acceptance. You see people where they are, and you work with them from there. Where they're at is where they're at. And bless their heart, you know?

My brother and sister are still very much a part of my life, and I'm grateful. But I've made it very clear. I flat out say to them, "No talk about religion or politics!" My safety comes first, and that involves staying calm and levelheaded.

Every day isn't easy. Derek and I still have our struggles, but thankfully using isn't one of them.

What Derek and I have now is heaven—almost literally. We recently acquired a pasture for our horse, and I can ride around the property. His name's Black Jack. I just call him Jack. He's like a big puppy dog. Really big. He's like sixteen or sixteen-plus hands. He's … wow—taller than me! And it's hard not to ride Black Jack, glance around, and marvel at how blessed I am to have this chance.

To me, this is what recovery—and hard reduction—is all about. It's good to have someone to talk to, and as some kind of anchor, spiritual or not. We need something that provides a sense of hope, not necessarily for the outcome. Because that's always going to be unknown. But in each moment, I can carry some kind of hope. If you know the Serenity Prayer, or know the Promises of the 12 Steps—I can't tell you how many times I've been in the rooms during a reading of those two, and just cried my eyes out. Because there is a lot of hope in that prayer. Because it shows us that the flip side of pain and hurt and misery is an unbelievable joy. That prayer holds a lot of hope in it. I don't do it alone. The biggest piece of that prayer reminds us to be safe. And never give up hope. Every day alive is another chance to get it right.

SUSAN OUSTERMAN

My journey into harm reduction began long before I knew the term existed, and yet, paradoxically, I did not always practice it. The deeply ingrained narrative of the War on Drugs created immense internal conflicts for me, especially as a mother. This narrative, which painted substance use as a moral failing or a criminal act, left me struggling to reconcile my love for my son with the fear and stigma associated with his substance use. I fought against the reality of his drug use, clinging to the hope that denial would somehow protect him. The conflict in my gut told a different story—a story of fear, love, and a desperate need for support.

At that time, the only support available to us as parents came from abstinence-based groups. These groups offered a single narrative: stop enabling your child and let them face the consequences of their choices. But what if those consequences were life-threatening? What if those choices were not truly choices at all, but rather the manifestation of an underlying, untreated mental health condition? My son was suffering, caught in the grips of substance use, and despite our best efforts, he was unable to access the care he so desperately needed.

The first time I consciously practiced harm reduction was a turning point for me. My son was staying in a hotel with his girlfriend, and they did not want us there. Despite our pleas, he refused to take naloxone with him, insisting that they were not using drugs. We knew better. The fear that something could go wrong was overwhelming, yet we had to find a way to support him without driving him further away. So, my daughter and I made a decision: we would leave him alone, as long as he checked in with us regularly. We spent that night in the car, parked in the hotel lot, with naloxone at the ready, prepared to break down the door if he didn't respond. We also left food and water outside his door, a small gesture of care in a situation where we felt so powerless.

This experience was my introduction to harm reduction, though I didn't recognize it as such at the time. It was simply an act of love—a way to protect my son without imposing judgments or expectations. It was a recognition that, while we could not control his choices, we could do everything in our power to keep him safe. I also knew that I needed to love and support my child just as any parent would if their child had a life-threatening condition.

For me, harm reduction is synonymous with unconditional love. It is about loving someone fully and without reservation, regardless of the circumstances they find themselves in. It is about doing everything possible to ensure their safety, while also respecting their autonomy. Harm reduction is not about condoning or condemning substance use; rather, it is about recognizing the humanity in each person and understanding that everyone deserves to be treated with dignity and compassion.

Harm reduction means meeting people where they are, without

projecting our expectations or judgments onto them. It is about creating a space where people feel safe to be themselves, where they can access the support they need without fear of stigma or rejection. This approach is not only life-saving but also life-affirming. It acknowledges that every person's journey is unique and that there is no one-size-fits-all solution to the challenges they face.

As parents, our instinct is to protect our children at all costs. In the face of the current overdose crisis, this instinct often manifests as fear—fear of losing our child, fear of what others will think, fear of the unknown. This fear is justified, given the devastating number of overdose deaths we have witnessed in recent years. However, it is crucial for parents to understand that substance use is not a moral failing or a simple choice. People use drugs for many reasons, often as a way to cope with trauma, mental illness, or other underlying issues. When substance use becomes problematic, it is usually a symptom of a deeper issue that needs to be addressed.

Expecting someone to simply stop using drugs without addressing the underlying causes is unrealistic and often counterproductive. In fact, for many people, especially those who have experienced trauma or who are dealing with complex mental health issues, the demand for immediate abstinence can be more harmful than helpful. When an individual is dependent on opioids, it can take up to eighteen months for their brain to regulate dopamine after they discontinue using. Without medication to assist during this period, returning to use is almost certain.

Harm reduction offers a different approach—one that recognizes the complexities of substance use and prioritizes the individual's safety and well-being over rigid expectations of sobriety. It is about providing people with the tools and support they need to reduce the risks associated with drug use, while also working to address the root causes of their substance use. For parents, this means shifting the focus from trying to control or fix their child's behavior to supporting them in a way that honors their autonomy and humanity. For example, access to sterile syringes may feel counterintuitive, but not having access is not going to stop them from using. I witnessed the impact of reusing syringes when my child contracted severe endocarditis and had to undergo open-heart surgery. You can cringe later, but ensure your child is being as safe as possible.

I envision a world where harm reduction is not just a practice, but a fundamental principle that guides our interactions with others. At its core, harm reduction is about rejecting assumptions, expectations, and judgments that can damage relationships and alienate individuals. It is about fostering an environment where people can live authentically, free from the fear of stigma or rejection.

In our society, there is often a rush to judgment—a tendency to categorize people based on their behaviors, their struggles, or their choices. This creates barriers to connection and understanding, making it difficult for people to feel accepted or supported. Harm reduction challenges these societal norms by promoting acceptance and compassion, even in the face of behaviors that are often stigmatized or misunderstood.

I would like to see harm reduction principles integrated into all aspects of our society, from healthcare to education, from law enforcement to community support systems. This would involve not only providing resources and support for those who use drugs but also creating a cultural shift that values empathy, understanding, and unconditional love. It would mean training healthcare providers, educators, and community leaders in harm reduction practices and ensuring that they have the tools and knowledge to support people in a way that is non-judgmental and compassionate.

Moreover, I believe that harm reduction should be a key component of our response to the overdose crisis. This includes expanding access to naloxone, providing safe consumption spaces, and ensuring that people who use drugs have access to healthcare, housing, and social services. But it also means addressing the root causes of substance use, such as trauma, poverty, and lack of access to mental healthcare. By taking a holistic approach to harm reduction, we can create a society where everyone has the opportunity to live a healthy, fulfilling life.

Harm reduction is more than just a set of practices—it is a philosophy of care and compassion that has the power to transform our society. My journey into harm reduction has been deeply personal, shaped by my love for my son and my desire to keep him safe. But it has also been a journey of learning and growth, as I have come to understand the importance of meeting people where they are, without judgment or expectation. I honor my son by practicing harm reduction in all aspects of my life.

Susan can be reached at http://www.vilomahfoundation.com

MEGHANN PERRY & SOPHIE PERRY-STEWART

Sophie: My mom and I were talking last night a bit about harm reduction, and I had never thought too much about it for myself. But I was thinking back, and I feel like I've been living a harm reduction type of lifestyle for a long time. And now that I'm older and I'm able to implement the tools that I've learned, my life centers around harm reduction. Harm reduction is a way of being for me. And I think it did start with a fear of using substances and losing control, but it morphed into, "How can I support myself in other areas," and "how can I do that for others as well?"

Harm reduction kind of started when I grew up. I had a DARE T-shirt when I was maybe 11 years old and I remember I was really scared of any substances at that point. That's when I learned that you could walk to the grocery store and people around you on the streets would be on drugs, but you don't know that and that made me fearful of people on drugs.

At that time, my harm reduction was abstinence, and then I fell into a group of friends my freshman year in high school. They smoked weed and did lots of other drugs, and I was very fearful for a long time. But that changed when I noticed how they would use but be the same loving, caring people. The fear subsided. I got to see both sides of drug use, or at least more than just one side. So, I started smoking weed, and I smoked weed for maybe six months before I was caught. And I really got caught. I got in a lot of trouble. It was a very emotional, embarrassing, shameful experience. So I was back to being abstinent again; once more the harm reduction was the abstinence.

Then later in high school I was seeing all these different types of friends, and we were going to the city, and everybody's doing all sorts of drugs I've never even heard of before. And I was curious again. I was also a lot older, and I had more independence. I also knew that I had to be a lot more mindful than my peers. So I wouldn't smoke weed at home or after school or before school. It was just for hanging out with my friends or seeing a movie with friends or something like that. Very social.

I realized that I needed to be mindful of my substance use because of my mom's history with substances. Thinking about that took up a large part of my brain. For a very long time, it was almost all I thought about. I believed that the worst thing that could happen to me was to become addicted, which is not true by the way.

Meghann: It's very interesting to listen to you talk about harm reduction, because it was the same thing with me: I didn't know I was practicing harm reduction. I never had the words or understood the principles of it but I practiced harm reduction the whole time I used substances. I was bleaching needles in the '90s, sharpening them on matchboxes. Going slow with new batches of heroin. And around the year 2000 we had an underground syringe delivery service in Portland, Maine, so I wasn't sharing needles with people. There were so many ways in which I was practicing harm reduction. I believe that when we look at people like me who survive injecting substances for long periods of time with high risk of fatality, harm reduction is largely behavioral. There's a lot of behavioral factors in action especially around using IV drugs more safely. I'd think about where I got my drugs from, asking around about the quality and potency; testing new brands by going slow/going small; being mindful of clean spoons, cotton and water; all of those kinds of positive behavioral things. And I had no idea *that* was harm reduction. I was just trying to survive.

I came into recovery in an abstinence-based model. Abstinence was my pathway. And I was "all in." We all lived that abstinence, which was the only option at the time. I lost custody of Sophie for six years, from ages four to ten, but I got her back. I didn't begin my abstinence until after I got her back. That was the last piece that I needed to say, "I can't ever use again, because I don't want to lose this kid." I had just gotten this kid back and so I was absolutely committed to an abstinence-based lifestyle as I believed that was the only way I could eliminate the risk of harm. I have always shared with Sophie about my life and my substance use challenges. We've been very honest with each other. She's learned much of what she knows about substances from me—up until the point when she was at an age to go and explore away from me, like she just shared. And my abstinence-only thinking ironically led me to deal badly with her using substances when I caught her with weed in her room. I freaked the F out. I walked out, in fact. I really lost it.

S: I remember. And that truly broke all the trust that we had spent so long building. It was this huge moment. I was 14, which is so young, and I was going into high school which means

425

pressure and I was already feeling that typical teen pressure and then you add this … this betrayal on my part, and it had a huge impact on both of us.

M: Yeah, it did. And I did not handle it the way that I would today. Once I learned about harm reduction, I started to understand that people can have all different kinds of relationships with substances. Back then I knew that some people could use recreationally—but then there was me and everyone I knew in my abstinence-based community so it existed on a very clear binary. I also knew that there's a lot of practical strategies one can apply, ways of being and using drugs safer. But it changed everything when I became aware that drug use was on a spectrum between casual use and recreational use and problematic use. So today, I wouldn't have freaked out like I did. But then? I threatened her with, "If I catch you again, you're going to detox, and my friends work there and the Recovery High School is 15 minutes away!" She was grounded for a month, which wasn't how I parented. Usually, I was the kind of parent who said, "You make choices and you're going to get harmed by some of those choices. I'm here to help you navigate that." I gave Sophie a lot of freedom, and I don't regret that. That's not something that I think I did badly, but handling the situation when she was 14 and I caught her with weed? I did handle that badly because I didn't have a harm reduction outlook then. And now I've come to harm reduction more recently, in large part, because everyone's freaking dying! My friends have been dying since 1995 and so many before that, but not like this … not like this. This amount of daily and sustained loss of life is profoundly devastating. And so my outrage is at the failure of the abstinence-based treatment system, and our 12 Step community, which God bless them for so many things, but they are not picking up the pieces and filling in the gaps by adapting or accepting those for whom 12 Step is not the answer.

Honestly, Sophie's taught me a lot about harm reduction, because of her relationship to substances and because we've been talking pretty openly about drug use for years. Not that I think she's told me everything, nor should she. But we've had *communication*. We've done a really good job of that in our relationship, so I've watched her, and she's talked to me about it, and that's all harm reduction.

S: I'm not sure how to phrase it, but I practiced a lot of harm reduction in my teens, just regarding other people using substances, being there with them when they used. I'm a very open person, and I found myself in a lot of, let's say, "stoner-type" friend groups. Actually, almost all my friend circles used all sorts of drugs and always have, but I never really went in for using substances much. I guess I stayed around them because I felt protective of my friends. I remember being eight or nine and my mom and I were visiting our place in Maine, which is where she would use I'm pretty sure, before we moved in together, and I'd overhear her talking about her friends who had overdosed. She'd get a phone call or something, and at that time, I knew that "overdose" always meant that they had passed away. It wasn't until I got older that I realized that you can survive an overdose.

M: That's a pretty profound thing to experience and live with as a child, Sophie. I wasn't even aware that you heard those phone calls, heard that friends had died by overdose. And that makes me really sad. I'm sorry that you had to experience that.

Another thing about all this is that the reality of death is very present for people with addiction and in recovery, and so that has never been far from the two of us. Getting Sophie back, she's had to hear about some of the worst that humanity has to offer because of the way we treat and address drug use and drug users. Just me talking with my partner at the time about friends that had died, or talking about it with other friends, and hearing the stories of being surrounded by death ... it's hard. Our village was partly at church in the early years, which, thank God, meant we had "healthy adults" in our circle. But our other village was entirely my friends in recovery, and the realities of what we talked about on a day-to-day basis was death, because we live with addiction right in our faces, especially once I started working in treatment. I started working as a recovery coach when Sophie was 14 and was bringing that home, and just having that reality to live in is hard. Add growing up knowing that your parent is also one of those people who could return to using drugs and die, that fear and how that impacts your own fear around your own substance use is something that we don't hear about nearly enough. Who is talking about the impact of that on our kids?

S: I didn't think about that. I don't have a whole lot of outlets to talk about recovery either. And I've realized that a lot of what keeps me—and kept me—from using a lot of substances is the fear of putting my mom through that again, for her to have to go back to those spaces. I didn't want to do that to her. It's hard, because I look at my mom and I know the things that she's been through, and to me they sound very challenging and horrible, but that was not enough to stop me because I have seen her being healthy since I was ten and that conflicts with the idea of her suffering so badly with substance use. I guess it makes me forget how bad it could be. It's hard to say that.

I think when I look at my mom and she's okay, I definitely see there is also hope. But it was the fear of her seeing me have a problem with substances, how hard that would be, that kept me from using a lot. Even more than that, though, my bigger fear wasn't that *I* would get into trouble for using substances but that it might bring *her* right back to drug use.

M: Wow, that's a lot to carry, Sophie.

S: Yeah, it is. And it's something I don't think I ever thought to tell you. Wow, this *is* a lot. Things are coming up that I didn't expect to come up. So this is good.

One of the things I've thought about is what you could have done differently when you caught me with cannabis. I don't want to say an intervention necessarily but I think really stopping everything and getting to the root my using weed would've helped. Asking the question, like, *why* was I using it? But I also understand that you were acting out of fear and I have no resentment now, though I did at the time. But now looking back, 14 is young, though at the time I thought I was grown. I thought I was old enough to make this choice. But I think that if my mom had stepped into my life more, given me a bit more structure—I just had so much freedom, so much space to do what I wanted and to form unhealthy habits—that would've made a difference. I smoked weed at first because I was curious, and then because it helped me go to sleep. I hate to say this, but she would go to a 12 Step meeting and I would smoke and be asleep by the time she got home.

I needed less freedom, but I also think that's tricky. You know what? I just realized that what I needed was safety. I needed safety in that situation. And instead, I lost my mom, and I was grounded, and it was freshman year; I already didn't have a lot of friends. So I decided to shave my head. Weird choice but it was something I could control.

M: I'm really sorry I did not give that safety to you.

S: I was just so isolated and I needed my mom.

M: And I was less than four years into recovery. For me, in that moment of finding your weed, I lost my mind because I was holding drugs in my hands for the first time in four years. And it was some good-looking weed!

S: You know I remember when you came into my room that night, you just yelled at me the whole time. And here I was sitting in my room thinking that I could gain your trust back if I just gave you the weed and my smoking pipe. I was making a bid for a connection with you. But boy did that backfire. Giving you the weed and pipe made everything so much worse. And so it killed me twice.

M: I'm not in any way defending how I behaved; I really, really wish I had handled it differently. But I want to share that when Sophie handed me the pipe and weed, it broke me. I was *terrified* to have drugs in my possession. I was at a place in my recovery where holding drugs, being around drugs, that was "to my bones" terror. What happened as a result of that fear when she came out of her room and handed me the pipe and the weed, is that I looked at it and I literally ran.

S: She didn't say a word, nothing.

M: I didn't say anything to Sophie. I grabbed the weed, grabbed the car keys, and ran out the door. I drove the car down the street and threw everything in a dumpster and sobbed. And that response from me came 100% from fear of my own addiction coming back; that was me being afraid for my recovery. And then, after all that, I think I was just really in shock. I wish that I could have connected with her and been there with her and for her, but as with so many other aspects of our relationship and my parenting, I was barely managing my own shit. That wasn't fair to Sophie at all, but it's the reality of our whole time together then. Living together was about me trying to hang on. And thinking how I wasn't even in abstinence-based recovery when I got you back. I had built up so many positive things in my life but still binging. So unfortunately, Sophie bore the brunt of me barely being able to be alive. I laugh because it sounds absurd but it's also not funny at all. These are the really deep realities of being a parent with problematic substance use, in or out of its resolution, and a teenager trying to figure out how to be her own person when my problems and my stuff is just so huge. I took up all the space in our lives for a while. It was just me trying to be in recovery and trying to take care of my trauma and all of that, but it wasn't fair to you, Sophie, at all.

S: And now looking back, I wonder why it didn't hit me until I gave her the weed, what that meant for her to have it, to hold it. When I gave her the weed, *that* was when I realized "Oh shit, I'm in trouble. Oh shit, what have I done?" I realized at that moment that *she* could be in trouble. And then I realized that if she's in trouble, *I'm* in trouble. So when she left, I was thinking, "What's gonna happen with our lives now?" I was scared, wondering if she's going to get caught up in using again because then she'll lose me again; I'll lose her again.

M: I want to know more about how you developed a healthy relationship with substances, Sophie, with all this chaos going on, because I know you're not completely substance free. You're managing what would be considered moderation or practicing harm reduction. What do you think makes the difference for you to be able to have a healthy relationship with substances and not a problematic one?

S: I think it's just ingrained in me to be mindful of all my habits. So anything that I'm doing consistently, I've learned to be mindful about because I also learned that anyone can be addicted to anything. I learned that at a young age. I developed a really unhealthy relationship with food. Coming out of that was kind of my start into harm reduction. I had to learn how to eat better. While I've been drunk before and I do drink occasionally now, the reason that I don't drink consistently or drink a lot is because I don't like how it makes me feel when I do that. I'll have a drink at dinner or something like that, and that feels good, but I know that if I have two drinks, I'm not going to feel good. And then drinking is pointless. I do take mushrooms though occasionally, but again, it's such a big feeling and I don't always want to feel that.

M: I think you partly just nailed the difference between you and me by saying it's such a big feeling that you don't want to feel that feeling all the time. I do. If it feels good, I want a lot more, still, whether it's food or sex or substances.

S: I've had days when it's a Saturday and I'll smoke weed in the morning and I'm so chill right then. But then I feel like crap the rest of the day. I know how good I feel sober, and I love being the designated driver, I love being coherent, I love being safe. I love feeling like me. And I also think that when I use substances, I'm not as in tune with other people: I'm not as a good friend or a guest, or there's that little layer of "me, me, me" and when I notice that, it hurts me.

While we've been talking, one thing I've realized about harm reduction is that it's personal to each person. I really think harm reduction is "how can you show up best for yourself and your community? What are the steps for you to be the best person you can be for you?" Then I also realize that if I'm being the best I can for *me* then I'm also going to be the best person for others in my community. So I just keep coming back to how harm reduction is just so personal—and it's situational, it's fluid. It's fluid for people throughout their lives and it's different for every person. So I think harm reduction is really just finding out what your personal goals or values are and focusing on how to get them.

M: I think it's similar in that it's a way of living my life so that my actions cause the least harm to myself and others. It's about being a good member of the community. It's about taking care of myself and taking care of other people. So no matter what it is that needs to be done, no matter what it looks like to take care of other people, that's what we need to do. Regardless of what that person's choices or circumstances are, whatever they're compelled to do for any number of different reasons, harm reduction is just saying, "Listen, we're all just trying to live by our values, reach our goals and be in community with one another." I think that harm reduction is rarely selfish, and I agree with Sophie that it's very fluid throughout life. What harm reduction looked like for me when I was using meant things like never cutting the drugs that I sold to other people. Never. It was important to me that I measured it out and you got the amount of the drug that you thought you were getting because I didn't want you to be harmed by what I was selling you. I also practiced harm reduction strategies with the drugs that I was using. Like I mentioned before, being careful and measuring and testing drugs before I used them, not sharing needles and other safer practices meant I was less likely to cause harm in my drug-user community. Today it's different since I no longer use those substances. But I think Sophie really nailed it by saying that it's just about how we are with one another and trying not to cause harm.

S: You know, it's really hard for me to relate because I'm *not* having a hard time thinking about what harm reduction is, because I feel like I've been living and thinking about harm reduction my whole life. I don't see the side against harm reduction very much, which is something I probably need to open my eyes to, just to understand where those folks are coming from. For instance, why *wouldn't* they want safe consumption sites? I can't wrap my head around that thinking, of being against safe consumption sites. So, I do think harm reduction really is about community, and how we can show up best for our community members. I also think that even if you're not practicing harm reduction for yourself, you can still practice it with other people.

M: Absolutely. I didn't get into harm reduction work until a bit into my own abstinence—and not that I don't practice harm reduction in other areas of my life, but when it comes to substances, I say that for me, abstinence is currently my harm reduction: I had to fully stop, there is no in-between for me. It was clearly profoundly problematic. I really like the way you talked about harm reduction though, Sophie, as just simply a way of being who you are. I appreciate that a lot and it's almost like this beautiful sort of childlike sense of thinking: "What do you mean you can't get behind a safe consumption site? We're going to kill people by not having those and we need to help them be safe." And it's not to "save" them to get somewhere that others have decided they should be, but it's definitely helping folks be in a place where they can make another choice if they want to. We should take care of each other and in part that looks like providing a safe space for folks to use their drug of choice; it looks like providing them with clean, sterile using equipment. We're giving them a space, a place, a product, an item of policy, whatever it is that takes care of them without wanting or feeling the need to change them. We do see a lot of people suffering profoundly with substance use or untreated mental health challenges, or in other challenging circumstances as a result and many of us wish things could be different for them, absolutely. But what *I wish* for someone else is not reducing harm, and it's sure not taking care of them. It's putting something of mine on to them and that doesn't align with human rights. Like the criminal justice system, which is mainly about incarcerating people—there's literally nothing in that system that's about caring for people.

S: I guess people just don't understand what harm reduction is really about. I mean, we have harm reduction around us all the time, we just don't acknowledge it or understand it. We also don't call it that. I wish people could see that harm reduction is so easy; it's right in front of you. It's so easy to practice harm reduction because we're already doing it in a lot of other areas. In fact, maybe in all other areas of our life. So why is it so hard to think about when it comes to substances? People need to understand that harm reduction actually brings you closer, not only to people you love but also to your community. It makes you a much more involved community member. It forces you to really see the people around you. It also makes you look at yourself and where you could be treating yourself better. I think it's very intimate. I also think that the reward is great.

M: You may have hit on something, Sophie. I wonder if that's part of what keeps people away from harm reduction, that fear of intimacy. The fear of having to look at myself, the fear of getting closer to folks that are involved in this risky behavior that scares the shit out of me. Wow, I am so in love with what you just brought! It *is* about intimacy and it *is* about love. We say it all the time, right? "Harm reduction is love." We say the word but I think that intimacy piece is what makes me really realize the deeper connection to how hard it can be to love us drug users up close when we use substances problematically, or have untreated mental health challenges. Each of those things separately are a lot and for some they intersect, which makes us even harder to love. Loving us up close can be incredibly painful and challenging, and harm reduction asks us to love up close. I think that's really scary for a lot of people. We know how hard it is to care that much, and loving someone up close while watching them struggle so much with life ... well it can be too much. I think that the arguments against harm reduction are at least in part because we would have to be intimate with that struggle or that person. We know people are suffering and in pain because of the challenges they're facing. And you know what? That's when we need to come back to the idea of self-care, what I think of as the harm reduction strategy for ourselves as individuals who care for folks. How close can I be? What is my acceptable level of intimacy, depth, and ability to provide harm reduction to people? How up close can I love them right now?

I'm thinking of an example from my and Sophie's life. I had a partner for eight years that I met while using and then we got into recovery together. Sophie came back to me four years into our relationship. So he was her stepfather for four years before the relationship ended and he left. He's currently incarcerated, facing a long prison sentence for trafficking, and I have not written to him. I haven't talked to him. I've sent a little bit of money through Sophie and that's all. But Sophie has talked to him regularly. She pays to make it possible for him to text her and email her. They've talked on the phone. She sends money. She's been a huge support for him. And I don't know what the malfunction is, but I can't do it. I cannot bring myself to have a loving relationship with him, even though I love him deeply. He's a phenomenal human who hasn't found a path to healthier living yet. I've been trying to figure out why I can't even just write to him and I think we might have just discovered the reason: That it is so painful for me to try to love him up close knowing what we went through as co-defendants in a previous trafficking case and the years that we used together. He's still living that trauma and I can't face going back to it. He's still in the same fight we were both in 15 years ago. And I just can't face that pain, or I can't love him that close up. It's too intimate.

I also think this is an important aspect of harm reduction and of taking care of each other that we don't talk about enough. I think often when we talk about it, we only talk about it in anger: "This is my boundary and I have to push you away!" Why can we push people we love away in anger but we can't have a gentle, intimate, loving conversation with them that says, "You're breaking my heart and I can't be with you right now?"

S: I think it's interesting that the only real experiences I have now is with people that are using substances in a way that is harmful to them. Growing up, I was a very open person who would talk to everybody. There I was in the winter, handing out hats and socks and things like that to folks living outside. But now I've had some experiences in my life and in the city and am too scared to talk to anybody no matter who they are. It's interesting how me practicing harm reduction for myself right now doesn't allow me to be there for others in the same way that I used to. I'm not able to have that intimacy, I'm not able to see them the same way right now. And I'm sitting here wondering why that is, why my fear is greater than my care for others. And I'm not sure, but I'm a little saddened by that.

M: I think compassion is what you have, Sophie. Compassion is what you've always had—very, very, very big compassion, which made you talk to and connect with everybody. We always did things like serving Thanksgiving meals at the shelter together. Or when I was in rehab and you'd come and stay for the weekend and you loved all the people there, even though they did things that other people thought were bad.

S: Like swearing, ha-ha!

M: You were so loving towards them. But we get compassion fatigue, and you live in the city now. You're surrounded by hopelessness and despair all the time, and it's hard to care up close and individually when it's just always, always, always, there; you're presented with it all the time. It's exhausting.

I do think you hit on something really significant about self-care and our own harm reduction. It's important that we recognize where our compassion for others ends and where our compassion for ourselves or self-care and our own harm reduction begins. And maybe this fatigue is what some folks are going through when they say they're against harm reduction, especially those who have experienced problematic use themselves and been around that pain for decades or even the majority of their lives. But I have to say this: I *really* wish people would get out of the way of those of us willing to work in harm reduction, those of us who are willing to be intimate, willing to love and support folks who use drugs. If it's not for you, if you're not the one who is going to go and fight to get safe consumption sites opened, if it's not for you to go and do street outreach, if it's not for you to be a clinician working with people who use drugs, just don't get in the way of those of us who will. Please just don't get in the way. Because if you do care about the community, if you really do care about people regardless of your beliefs about "right" and "wrong," you would see that we're doing an important job, we're playing an important role in the ecosystem, a role that's desperately needed. Of course I wish folks could see all the good that is harm reduction, all of the ways in which we take care of each other that are good. And none of those ways need to have a moral value attached to them besides just caring about one another. But it's hard to be compassionate when you're scared and I think a lot of people are scared of drug users, and scared their own health or recovery will be threatened by supporting drug users. But we have to love, to be intimate with each other anyway. That's the only way through all of this—for some of us to love really, really up close, and for the rest of us not to stand in the way.

Meghann and Sophie can be reached at
meghann@meghannperry.com
https://www.meghannperry.com
sophiegps@hotmail.com

TORI MILLER

I had always been sensitive to alcohol and drugs. I had never really even drunk much, never used any recreational drugs. Then I met someone who used. I thought that that would be a deal breaker for me. But at the time, he was very open to going to a methadone clinic. And I was very supportive. We hear about people going into rehabs and we've supportive. But with methadone, we were able to live together through that process. I'll forever be thankful for all that time together.

Sadly, we're no longer together. He actually passed away. But we had several years. With methadone and later suboxone, he was able to have contact with his children. We enjoyed several years before passed, remaining friends after we weren't a couple. I'm very grateful to methadone and suboxone for that. Those medications were my introduction to harm reduction.

There was definitely a stigma, especially for him. And so it was something he was having to fight. Personally, I felt it seemed like the natural thing to do. And then after, once we were together, I met one of his closest friends. The two of them had been in prison together, both in drug-related issues. And so

I became close friends with his friend as well. And the friend was in drug court. Unfortunately, he died of an overdose.

Shortly after leaving jail and going to rehab, in 2012, I became officially introduced to harm reduction.

At first, for me, it was just agreeing with the principles like methadone and other harm-saving practices. It came natural to me—it came natural to respect what was right for each *individual*. Autonomy, respect, honoring the person—for me, these are the cornerstones of harm reduction.

After these personal losses, I attended the 2012 Southeastern Harm Reduction Convention. I was just blown away! It was very soon after my husband died. And then, at that conference, we learn about how Naloxone and the Good Samaritan laws were being used in North Carolina. At the conference, we're learning *two different things* that could have saved our friends' lives! The exposure at the that conference led to the creation of similar groups and laws here in Georgia.

That was how I became more exposed to some of the people working in harm reduction, learning more of the principles.

In my case, I developed some health issues soon after. Sadly, I wasn't able to participate in the process as much as I'd like.

I think harm reduction is more than narrowly defined strategies; harm reduction is *any time* you can reduce the harms of drug use. A big part of this centers around respect for the drug user, which includes trusting them to make the decisions for themselves.

Wth all of the evidence proving the effectiveness of methadone and suboxone, I'm frustrated that the stigma around those two continue. I wish we were there—now. I want to see people have access to all of those both, and the comfort that comes with knowing that.

It's frustrating to see the financial barriers for people. It's frustrating that people have to go to the clinic for methadone. I would like to see easier access. If we eliminate those barriers, it'd be more accepted. I know so many people who benefited from those medications in the past, and could in the future, too. That was why I wanted to participate in this (new edition of *Kicking and Screaming*), to talk about how these medications have helped the people I care about. And not only with my then-husband—I have several other friends who had benefited from those medications. In addition to increased access, I'd like to see this issue of drug use and resulting behaviors moved out of the criminal courts. It needs to be treated for the social issue it truly is.

Like the cases of my ex-husband and other friends, I know too many people caught up in this. Users have so many arrests, so many interactions with law enforcement, jail stays while trying to go through withdrawal—hard time in prison. All the trauma makes it more difficult to get the life they want.

Here in Georgia, we *are* making progress. I wish it was more. But we do have Naloxone access now, and there's starting to be *some* syringe exchange services. Not as many as I would like. But it's a start.

I feel that AA has permeated our culture so much—from the courts to cinema. It's just accepted. Drinking too much? Using too much? Go to AA! People don't realize there are other options, one of which is harm reduction.

Community is important. American culture values independence so much. Sometimes to the point of pathologizing connection with other people. This is the part AA gets right: bringing people together.

I just encourage more independent thinking.

Tori can be reached through
deedeestoutconsulting@gmail.com

INDEX

A

A Shot in the Dark 15

abscesses 95, 201, 208

abstinence 13, 14, 22, 23, 24, 26, 27, 28, 30, 31, 32, 66, 76, 84, 90, 91, 110, 113, 114, 115, 147, 148, 154, 155, 157, 160, 161, 166, 173, 175, 185, 192, 197, 198, 199, 200, 201, 204, 220, 221, 233, 234, 237, 238, 240, 245, 246, 248, 249, 271, 278, 279, 280, 281, 282, 285, 296, 297, 301, 307, 308, 309, 310, 312, 313, 314, 318, 326, 335, 348, 356, 362, 364, 387, 388, 389, 391, 392, 393, 401, 402, 403, 404, 405, 406, 418, 420, 424, 425, 426, 427, 432, 435

abstinence violation effect (AVE) 27

abuse 98, 120, 142, 148, 149, 165, 186, 222, 233, 268, 269, 270, 286, 290, 326, 328, 329, 411

access to care 125

Access Works 221

accountability 26

ACOA 356

ACT UP 112, 207

active users 183

acupuncture 47

addict 47, 64, 75, 106, 107, 125, 131, 132, 168, 175, 207, 267, 268, 270, 313, 345, 356, 374, 375, 381, 411, 412

addicted 13, 49, 71, 94, 101, 204, 282, 285, 321, 358, 360, 396, 425, 433

addiction 10, 11, 26, 36, 37, 38, 63, 64, 65, 71, 77, 86, 94, 99, 107, 130, 149, 150, 155, 157, 164, 169, 186, 240, 244, 248, 251, 253, 254, 255, 257, 258, 279, 280, 281, 283, 284, 286, 289, 290, 291, 292, 302, 303, 304, 317, 318, 321, 323, 324, 326, 354, 355, 356, 357, 358, 359, 363, 364, 366, 367, 368, 371, 373, 375, 379, 382, 388, 392, 393, 394, 399, 401, 403, 406, 410, 411, 412, 414,

429, 432

addiction treatment 10, 204, 233, 254, 256, 257, 284, 355, 356, 359, 360, 366, 371, 373, 375

addictive 203, 278, 285, 287

addictive behaviors 243, 244, 245, 247, 275, 284, 317, 318, 321, 324, 325, 326, 328

Addictive Behaviors Model 321

addictive disorder 257

addictive personality 396

adolescent 305, 387, 388

adulteration 139, 140

advice 26, 84, 93, 94, 174, 230, 236, 239, 281, 302, 362, 365, 383

advocacy 80, 81, 82, 83, 84, 86, 173, 202, 303, 304, 305, 313

African 47, 51, 54

AIDS 48, 49, 50, 64, 67, 79, 80, 83, 94, 95, 139, 166, 181, 207, 231, 307, 308, 312, 345, 348

AIDS Benefits Counselors (ABC) 79

Air Force 99

Albuquerque 83, 274,

Al-Anon 94, 357, 374,

alcohol 11, 20, 23, 27, 29, 31, 32, 33, 37, 46, 54, 66, 67, 73, 75, 76, 93, 95, 107, 121, 143, 147, 168, 176, 185, 186, 187, 197, 201, 203, 204, 218, 219, 220, 221, 223, 225, 235, 247, 248, 249, 259, 260, 261, 262, 264, 274, 275, 311, 317, 318, 319, 320, 321, 322, 323, 324, 325, 327, 329, 339, 342, 354, 356, 358, 361, 362, 392, 395, 396, 398, 399, 410, 442

alcohol harm reduction 221

Alcohol Skills Training Program (ASTP) 322

alcohol use disorder (AUD) 37, 218, 312

alcoholic 66, 219, 235, 248, 321, 325, 329, 356, 409

Alcoholics Anonymous (AA) 27, 28, 38, 43, 65, 66, 67, 68, 72, 73, 75, 76, 77, 93, 97, 101, 102, 103, 104, 106, 108, 112, 114, 132, 148, 175, 177, 211, 218, 219, 220, 222, 237, 247, 263, 267, 270, 271, 331, 332, 339, 356, 358, 401, 409, 444, 445

alcoholism 37, 94, 186, 274, 275, 317, 321, 362, 399

Alexander, Michelle 156

alternatives 77, 132, 156, 184, 199, 225, 238, 240, 241, 318, 375

ambivalence 34, 236, 287, 336, 393,

Amsterdam 139

anarchists 140

Anderson, Kenneth 16, 217-223, 335

anger 11, 78, 176, 211, 229, 246, 290, 303, 364, 372, 381, 399, 438

Anslinger, Harry 54, 55, 58, 59

antidepressants 148, 409

anxiety 14, 35, 36, 80, 98, 100, 178, 239, 243, 260, 286, 287, 322, 352, 373, 376, 378, 403

Arapahoe House 260, 261

Argentina 80

Arizona 83,

arrest 55, 120, 141, 144, 187, 209,

304, 319, 372, 401, 412, 444

Art of Loving, The 285

Ashford, Robert 123, 124

attachment theory 357, 383

autonomy 23, 26, 87, 91, 132, 134, 141, 197, 200, 227, 318, 335, 336, 419, 421, 443

aversion therapy 325

B

baby steps 35, 398, 414

Baker, Philip 225-232

Baltimore 83, 352

BASICS 323

Baum, Dan 55

Bear, Daniel 19

Beattie, Melody 356, 373, 374, 375, 376

Beck, Aaron 324

behavioral addictions 324

Behavioral Alcohol Research Laboratory 321

behavioral change 240

behavioral health 102, 104, 114, 130, 140, 269, 271

behavioral self-control 275,

benefits 52, 53, 63, 75, 76, 79, 113, 142, 146, 157, 179, 183, 198, 253, 264, 284, 294, 295, 332, 337, 339, 444

Berkeley 139, 410

Berkeley Needle Exchange 137

Big Book 93, 102, 104, 105, 106,

107, 271, 358,

Big Pharma 234

Bigg, Dan 16, 42, 59, 90, 120, 217

biopsychosocial 104, 324, 325

BIPOC 45, 49

bipolar disorder 260, 302

bisexual 94,

Black 46, 48, 49, 50, 51, 52, 53, 54, 55, 56, 57, 79, 82, 84, 85, 86, 91, 100, 155, 156, 213, 307, 337

black and white 220, 361, 376, 391, 404

Black, Claudia 356

Black Harm Reduction Network (BHRN) 48

Black Panthers 47, 203

bleach 153, 425

blow 118

boofing 183

boosting 101

Boston 112, 186, 237, 293, 294, 295

Boston City Hospital 293

Boston Medical Center 295

boundaries 262, 265, 301, 375, 376, 388, 389, 438

Bourassa, Brian 63-69

brain disease 37, 240, 279

brief intervention 274, 322

British Columbia 115, 273

Brooklyn 192

Brown 57, 79, 82, 85, 86, 155, 213

Brown, Mike 173-179

Buddha 81, 187

Buddhism 81, 181, 184, 185, 187, 188

Bukowski, Charles 184

buprenorphine (bupe) 44, 83, 92, 143, 157, 271

Burns, David 324

Burns, Gretchen 303

Butler, Adam 208

C

Cali-sober 23, 28

California 79, 83, 166, 181, 186, 225, 261

cannabis 92, 173, 176, 177, 199, 201, 305, 323, 329, 337, 347, 378, 430

capacity building 82, 84

Castro 68

Caucasian 201

Caudill, Barry 273, 274

Celebrate Recovery 268

Center for Strength-Based Strategies 233

chairwork 283, 285, 286, 287, 288, 289, 291, 292

chaos 122, 164, 208, 299, 397, 432

chaotic use 23, 192, 204, 336, 374, 381, 395, 405

character defects 318, 339, 340, 396

chauvinism 115, 142

Chavez, Maria 84

Chicago Recovery Alliance (CRA) 16, 42, 59

child/children 9, 10, 47, 48, 94, 96, 99, 110, 138, 192, 230, 245, 287, 290, 319, 320, 340, 341, 353, 356, 361, 362, 366, 373, 374, 378, 383, 389, 391, 392, 393, 394, 396, 399, 405, 418, 419, 420, 421, 428, 435, 442

China White 118

chipping 100, 413

Chocolate Chip Effect 352

choice 28, 30, 31, 110, 129, 133, 143, 146, 157, 161, 164, 167, 188, 230, 237, 238, 254, 278, 297, 306, 327, 348, 352, 353, 374, 388, 410, 418, 419, 420, 421, 427, 430, 431, 434, 436

Choudry, Tripti 15, 44

Christ 187, 380, 415

Christian 73, 74, 415

chronic 10, 37, 68, 201, 279, 319

chronic pain 55, 199, 282, 313

cigarettes 175, 176,

Clark, Michael 233-241

class 25, 41, 46, 49, 75, 117, 147, 148, 186, 197, 201, 202, 207, 209, 213, 264, 279, 280, 333, 356, 366, 405

classism 213

clean and sober 364, 396

clean needles 19, 49, 50, 52, 75, 148, 154

Cleveland 102,

client-centered 229, 235, 236, 237,

264, 318, 359

Clifasefi, Seema 13, 246

Clifford, Joe 15, 71-78

co-occurring disorders 259, 302

cocaine 73, 201, 217, 346, 348, 402

Cocaine Anonymous 401

Codependent No More 373, 376

codependency 311, 358, 360, 361, 363, 369, 371, 372, 373, 374, 375, 376, 380, 381, 411

cognitive behavioral therapy (CBT) 245, 248, 251, 279, 324, 325

cognitive dissonance 193

cold turkey 130, 335

collaboration 198, 283, 317

Collins, Susan 13, 18, 243-251

communication 75, 181, 186, 301, 311, 364, 365, 366, 368, 371, 376, 379, 407, 428

community 22, 24, 39, 48, 49, 50, 52, 53, 54, 56, 67, 73, 81, 82, 91, 92, 95, 102, 107, 108, 114, 123, 124, 130, 133, 140, 141, 156, 164, 168, 174, 179, 182, 183, 186, 193, 194, 202, 203, 209, 210, 211, 225, 247, 249, 257, 260, 265, 268, 271, 274, 275, 277, 297, 300, 302, 303, 312, 317, 322, 326, 328, 330, 335, 342, 361, 388, 391, 411, 421, 422, 427, 434, 435, 436, 440, 444

compassion 25, 26, 33, 35, 43, 72, 98, 108, 143, 165, 167, 170, 175, 194, 198, 208, 227, 228, 229, 230, 248, 254, 255, 256, 290, 291, 306, 313, 318, 327, 329, 336, 363, 383, 392, 399, 419, 421, 422, 439, 440

compassion fatigue 439

compulsion 291,

condoms 52, 90

Coney Island 192

confrontation 160, 181, 236, 239, 291, 313, 356, 362

connection 163, 175, 183, 193, 194, 195, 201, 260, 298, 375, 421, 431, 437, 445

consequences 21, 22, 33, 37, 95, 122, 200, 239, 247, 278, 299, 323, 326, 336, 357, 418

continuum 24, 27, 43, 200, 204, 250

controlled drinking 274, conversations 15, 22, 23, 37, 38, 40, 42, 50, 68, 75, 76, 85, 96, 112, 113, 118, 122, 138, 142, 144, 182, 186, 192, 193, 228, 230, 246, 248, 250, 270, 288, 311, 340, 346, 355, 359, 361, 362, 364, 367, 368, 378, 379, 388, 389, 438

coping 24, 34, 36, 178, 285, 287, 321, 322, 328, 340, 360, 363, 373, 381, 420

Correctional Service of Canada 326

corruption 176

counterfeit pills 139, 140

counterintuitive 280, 336, 421

couples 13, 18, 41, 356, 359, 360, 365, 366, 368, 369, 378, 379, 380, 382, 383, 384, 403, 406, 414, 442

courage 81, 123, 126, 193, 230,

Covid 82, 83, 174, 183, 233, 399

crack 49, 52, 107, 183, 201

crack baby 52

crack house 101

CRAFT 328, 330, 388, 391, 392

criminal justice 230, 237, 245, 436

Crowder, Don 46

Cullen, Denise 303

cult 331

D

DanceSafe 137, 139, 140, 141, 144

DARE 176, 179, 405, 424

Dead Set on Living 366, 369

decriminalization 115, 144, 399

defund the police 82

degradation 150

dehumanizing 194, 311, 342

demonizing 146, 335

denial 31, 35, 114, 418

Denning, Patt 20, 43, 261, 285, 302, 328, 361, 363, 369, 383

Denver 259, 260

depressant 259

depression 100, 148, 218, 243, 255, 259, 260, 286

deprogramming 119, 134,

disconnection 257

designated driver 433

despair 95, 119, 439

destigmatize 110

destructive 165, 187, 341, 342, 343, 347, 395

detox 67, 102, 103, 104, 220, 374, 427

dharma 187

Dharma Punks 187

diagnosis 10, 79, 229, 248, 260, 269, 307, 311, 312, 319, 360, 375, 376

dialectical behavioral therapy (DBT) 305

dialogue 67, 68, 186, 213, 287, 288, 292

dignity 158, 164, 193, 198, 208, 263, 419

discrimination 21, 25, 51, 91, 119

disease 22, 37, 38, 50, 51, 75, 107, 114, 153, 200, 240, 279, 293, 294, 297, 307, 317, 318, 321, 326, 339, 340, 348, 354, 356, 358

disempowerment 325

distress 149, 254, 283, 290, 340, 362, 363

doctors 46, 51, 55, 72, 82, 93, 107, 108, 126, 127, 143, 144, 148, 174, 235, 248, 251, 357, 358, 377, 409

domestic violence 165

dope 149, 270, 293

dope sick 100

Drinker's Checkup 276, 322, 323

drinking 10, 31, 37, 65, 66, 67, 73, 76, 77, 93, 122, 175, 217, 218, 219, 220, 221, 223, 247, 248, 259, 260, 273, 274, 276, 278, 279, 318, 319, 321, 322, 323, 337, 356, 361, 396, 409, 411, 415, 433, 444

Drop the Label 106, 107, 108

drug checking 109, 114, 139, 140, 143, 144

drug court 234, 238, 240, 443

drug dealer 11, 165, 294

Drug Enforcement Administration (DEA) 54, 55, 138, 157, 328

drug laws 21, 56, 199, 202,

drug policy 21, 22, 118, 121, 122, 155, 156, 303, 304, 397

Drug Policy Alliance (DPA) 22, 53, 302

drug-related harms 87

Drug, Set, Setting 364

drug supply 82, 297

drug testing strips 19

drug tests 31, 198, 402

Drug Use for Grownups 342

drug user health 82

drug-user organizing 209

drug users union 231

Drug War. See War on Drugs

drunk 31, 72, 76, 218, 219, 220, 261, 433, 442

drunk driving 84

DSM 34, 200, 229, 248, 263, 360

dual diagnosis. See co-occurring disorders

Dutch 139

DWI 276

dysfunctional 356

E

East Harlem 48

Eau Claire 217

ecstasy 137, 138, 139, 141

Edina 220

Education Development Center 295

Ehrlichman, John 55

EMDR 415

emotional connection 375

empathy 77, 86, 318, 327, 414, 422

empowerment 306, 325,

enabling 154, 168, 174, 213, 255, 298, 345, 371, 372, 373, 377, 378, 379, 380, 388, 403, 411, 418

endocarditis 421

endorphin 158, 358

Ensure 65

environment 10, 13, 23, 26, 93, 168, 227, 230, 256, 257, 421

equity 83, 87, 121, 125, 133, 195

Erowid 109

ethical 35, 256, 342, 343

Europe 54, 273

European 201

evidence-based 106, 175, 236, 250, 263, 318, 323, 326, 400

exile 112

experimentation 118, 281

F

Face to Face 166, 167, 169

Facebook 110, 222

family 10, 13, 29, 33, 34, 38, 46, 51, 79, 90, 94, 95, 98, 99, 103, 178, 188, 207, 209, 243, 244, 247, 250, 253, 256, 257, 270, 293, 302, 305, 330, 351, 353-369, 371, 374, 376, 378,

380, 381, 383, 388, 394, 397, 400, 406, 411

father 75, 93, 94, 97, 98, 99, 118, 165, 166, 243

Favaro, Jamie 173

fear 50, 54, 64, 100, 134, 144, 282, 290, 332, 362, 365, 371, 394, 399, 407, 409, 414, 418, 419, 420, 421, 424, 425, 429, 430, 431, 432, 437, 439

Federal Bureau of Narcotics 54, 58

Federal Bureau of Prisons 326

fentanyl 96, 140, 143, 144, 145, 146, 158, 169, 204, 233, 234, 238, 271, 352

fentanyl test strips 144, 145, 146, 169, 352

Fernandez, Jennifer 253-258

first person 289,

fixing reflex 236

flexibility 188, 311

food 10, 19, 63, 77, 108, 140, 169, 199, 245, 319, 388, 419, 433

Food Not Bombs 137, 140

Franskoviak, Perri 253, 259-265

Frederique, Kassandra 53

freedom 86, 87, 133, 203, 222, 268, 283, 286, 289, 427, 430

Fromm, Erich 285

Fulgham, Robb 267-271

G

Garlington, Warren 274, 275

Gateway Foundation 117

gay 95, 139, 153, 312, 345

gender 204, 329

gender affirming care 202

genetics 187, 282

genuineness 239,

Gestalt 286

getting high 76, 102, 103, 158

Glide Harm Reduction 226, 231

goals 14, 26, 29, 30, 32, 35, 134, 155, 169, 182, 184, 200, 220, 223, 251, 284, 291, 313, 318, 359, 366, 374, 380, 387, 392, 405, 434

God 73, 75, 77, 157, 158, 194, 208, 211, 220, 222, 263, 323, 346, 396, 427, 429

Goethe, Johann 42, 351

Goffman, Erving 347

Good Samaritan Laws 304, 443

goth 138

Gottman Institute 379

government 36, 49, 50, 51, 139, 143, 157, 158, 199, 218, 348

grassroots 140, 141, 142, 229, 304

Grosso, Chris 366, 369

guilt 174, 201, 207, 339, 398, 402, 403

Guzman, Laura 79-87

H

habit 14, 185, 236, 322, 430, 433

Habitat for Humanity 268

Haight-Ashbury 139, 411

HAMS 16, 221, 222, 335

Hanna Somatics 415

Harm Reduction (book) 20, 36, 43, 44, 50, 58, 59

Harm Reduction Coalition (HRC) 21, 22, 47, 58, 83, 192, 209

Harm Reduction Psychotherapy (book) 20

harm reduction psychotherapy (HaRT; HRT) 12, 13, 14, 15, 20, 22, 23, 30, 32, 33, 35, 40, 41, 44, 253, 254, 255, 256, 257, 258, 261, 263, 283, 284, 285, 287, 288, 289, 292, 304, 305, 317, 318, 327, 328, 354, 355, 359, 361, 363, 366, 368, 369, 378, 382, 383,

Harm Reduction Therapy Center (HRTC) 20, 43, 253

Harm Reduction Training Institute (HRTI) 84

Harper's 55

Hart, Carl 205, 342

hate 11, 74, 85, 133, 184, 186, 188, 213, 281, 375, 381, 403, 430

Hawaii 67

healing 86, 139, 189, 191, 192, 193, 194, 197, 199, 258, 283, 286, 287, 290, 291, 313, 354, 400

healthcare 15, 22, 25, 43, 47, 48, 50, 51, 126, 143, 168, 186, 200, 203, 227, 248, 251, 264, 270, 421, 422

Healthcare for the Homeless (HCH) 82

healthcare industry 92

hegemony 113

helplessness 134, 325

Helton, Tracey 89-96

hep-C 64, 75, 95, 112, 182, 186, 191, 208

heroin 19, 42, 55, 73, 80, 90, 100, 101, 103, 118, 145, 163, 177, 199, 201, 207, 208, 210, 217, 239, 293, 297, 298, 299, 307, 346, 410, 425

Heroin Conference 90

heroin maintenance 143, 144, 145, 346, 348

Hester, Reid 273-278

high risk situations 325

Higher Power 73, 318

hitting bottom 85, 187, 335, 354, 372, 374

HIV 20, 48, 50, 64, 75, 80, 112, 139, 153, 155, 163, 166, 169, 179, 182, 186, 191, 293, 294, 295, 307, 347

holistic 13, 15, 113, 355, 359, 415, 422

Holland 346

home group 113, 114, 174

homeless 39, 63, 71, 73, 82, 83, 86, 89, 92, 112, 125, 138, 140, 149, 150, 218, 227, 230, 246, 295

Homeless Youth Alliance 226

honesty 36, 208, 239

hope 14, 15, 16, 42, 45, 75, 92, 96, 108, 123, 131, 132, 134, 170, 195, 210, 229, 239, 255, 279, 292, 296, 306, 342, 353, 355, 366, 368, 377, 381, 401, 416, 418, 430

hopelessness 131, 155, 362, 439

Horney, Karen 373

Horvath, Tom 303

housing 52, 63, 82, 83, 84, 85, 86, 91, 92, 115, 178, 200, 218, 249, 262, 422

Housing First 249

human rights 21, 54, 86, 87, 436

humanism 25

humiliation 160

humor 78, 333, 364

husband 75, 308, 356, 358, 361, 362, 397, 405, 443, 444

hygiene 108,

I

identity politics 337

illegal 54, 55, 201, 235, 327, 354

illicit 11, 15, 19, 24, 25, 47, 49, 52, 55, 93, 109, 203, 299, 328, 354, 379

imperialism 115

impending doom 100

In the Realm of Hungry Ghosts 302

incarceration 82, 245, 299, 399

incrementalism 26

individualism 26

inequality 48, 82, 156

infections 65, 95, 168, 297

injection 111, 159, 168, 170, 329

inpatient 164, 276,

instincts 32, 131, 396, 420

insurance 63, 92, 177, 264, 313, 361,

intimacy 40, 437, 439

integration 257, 289

Integrative Harm Reduction Psychotherapy 283

internet 154, 156, 157

intervention 22, 25, 26, 112, 226, 229, 231, 237, 249, 257, 274, 277, 322, 323, 412, 430

intoxication 322

intravenous 75, 111, 153

Invitation to Change (ITC) 391, 392

isolation 25, 96, 257, 394

IV drug use 49, 50, 64, 89, 101, 137, 140, 153, 173, 293, 426

J

Jaffe, Adi 279-282

jail 31, 33, 83, 90, 96, 102, 178, 186, 225, 230, 276, 299, 443, 444

Japan 217, 218

Jesus 77, 256, 415

Johnston, Kyle 97-108

Jones, Diane 80

judgment 33, 35, 64, 65, 77, 143, 146, 167, 193, 227, 256, 304, 310, 336, 347, 402, 419, 420, 421, 422

junkie 74, 94, 154, 188, 189, 329

Junkie Love 15, 71, 75

K

Kellogg, Scott 283-292, 303

Kelly, Michael 181-189

Kensington 125

kindness 72, 187, 188, 240, 372

Kinzly, Mark 120

Kishline, Audrey 219, 220

L

Lacks, Henrietta 51

Langis, Gary 112, 293-300

Latinx 47, 91,

laudanum 76

law enforcement 9, 225, 421, 444

law school 79, 118, 119

Leaders and Community Alternatives 225

learned helplessness 134

legal system 31, 176

legalization 76, 115, 156, 329, 348,

Lemire, Dean 123

lesbian 95, 312

Lessin, Barry 301-306

Lewis, Marc 18

LGBTQ 45, 48, 202

liberation 80, 115, 203, 292

LifeRing Secular Recovery 130, 133

limits 118, 219, 223, 355, 366, 367, 376, 383

literature 44, 65, 108, 150, 155, 268, 274

Little, Jeannie 20, 43, 84, 285, 302, 328, 383

Liverpool 49, 50, 345, 346, 348

Lord's Prayer 74

Los Angeles 181, 237

love 14, 38, 39, 42, 68, 77, 80, 81, 86, 94, 96, 133, 139, 165, 170, 173, 175, 185, 188, 193, 194, 195, 200, 201, 202, 210, 211, 226, 227, 239, 244, 256, 257, 258, 264, 284, 285, 286, 290, 311, 320, 323, 329, 336, 337, 347, 348, 355, 356, 367, 371, 375, 376, 380, 381, 383, 388, 392, 393, 396, 397, 400, 406, 418, 419, 422, 433, 436, 437, 438, 440

Love and Addiction 324

LSD 217, 402

M

Maine 382, 425, 428

major depression 255, 260

maladaptive 321, 360

Malcolm X Mental Health Center 259

mandatory 84, 115

marginalized 39, 47, 95, 199, 285

marijuana 55, 234, 235, 320

Marines 99

Marks, Don 346

Marlatt, G. Alan 20, 27, 35, 36, 38, 43, 44, 50, 58, 59, 248, 273, 274, 275, 317, 320

Marquis reagent 139

Marsh, Earle 358, 369

Marsh, Mickey 358

Maslow 199

mass incarceration. See incarceration

Massachusetts 112, 182, 183, 185,

207, 213

Mate, Gabor 200, 302, 366, 367, 368, 382

McVinney, Don 192

MDMA 138, 139

MDRI 345

Medi-Cal 79, 80, 269

Medicaid 277

Medicare 91, 264

medication assisted treatment (MAT) 40, 83, 175, 177, 233, 234

meditation 358

mental health 34, 37, 95, 106, 107, 140, 165, 178, 257, 259, 260, 261, 262, 263, 264, 268, 269, 301, 302, 308, 328, 361, 375, 379, 399, 418, 420, 422, 436, 437

mescaline 201

methadone 20, 77, 83, 90, 92, 143, 157, 166, 183, 202, 226, 271, 329, 345, 346, 395, 397, 413, 442, 443, 444

methamphetamine (meth) 65, 66, 67, 73, 80, 142, 163, 173, 177, 183, 279, 319, 358, 398

militarism 82

Miller, Tori 442-445

Miller, William 43, 236, 239, 274, 275, 276, 322, 324,

mindful 109, 425, 426, 433

Minneapolis 217, 219, 220, 221

Minnesota 39, 217,

Minnesota Model 356

misogyny 114

misuse 106, 107, 255, 270

moderate drinking 221, 274, 276, 278

moderation 20, 23, 93, 113, 219, 220, 221, 274, 282, 285, 288, 392, 433

Moderation Management 219, 221

Molina Health 277

monetization 113

money 46, 75, 96, 104, 119, 126, 144, 145, 165, 176, 212, 222, 228, 231, 264, 269, 277, 296, 298, 299, 312, 324, 397, 411, 438

Moore, Lisa 16, 38, 39, 53

moral model 317, 318, 320, 321

Moreno, Jacob 285

morphine 282

Morris, Terry 63

mortality 157

mother 75, 94, 95, 97, 98, 118, 178, 243, 248, 319, 351, 353, 398, 399, 418

motivation 24, 26, 31, 32, 99, 235, 236, 240, 330, 372, 391

motivational interviewing (MI) 54, 200, 210, 229, 236, 239, 245, 251, 279, 322, 333, 388

Motivational Interviewing (book) 43, 275

murder 82, 343

Murphy, Megan 166

mushrooms 320, 402, 433

mutual aid 32, 39, 115, 200

N

naloxone 22, 44, 90, 112, 120, 124, 144, 159, 173, 212, 304, 419, 422, 443, 444

Narcan 15, 19, 40, 44, 77, 105, 112, 169, 182, 183, 271, 297, 352, 353, 397

Narcotic and Drug Research Institute 49

Narcotics Anonymous (NA) 68, 73, 75, 90, 174, 175, 177, 267, 270

narrative 40, 102, 103, 153, 195, 203, 213, 289, 304, 312, 418

National Epidemiological Survey on Alcohol and Related Conditions (NESARC) 218

National Harm Reduction Coalition (NHRC). See Harm Reduction Coalition

National Healthcare for the Homeless 82

National Institute on Alcohol Abuse and Alcoholism (NIAAA) 37, 275,

National Institute on Drug Abuse (NIDA) 10, 279

Native 86

Natural Mind, The 324

needle exchange 19, 48, 49, 63, 89, 90, 111, 137, 139, 155, 159, 164, 166, 181, 182, 183, 208, 210, 211, 221, 222, 271, 294, 299, 300, 327, 329

negotiation 359, 360

Negron, Julia 303

neurodivergent 14

neuropathy 307

neuroplasticity 10, 18

neuroscience 18, 254, 279,

neurosis 373

Never Use Alone 173, 179

New England Prevention Alliance (NEPA) 300

New Jim Crow, The 156

New Mexico 274, 275, 276, 277,

New York City 20, 39, 47, 48, 49, 153, 181, 221, 222,

newcomers 105, 107, 148, 267,

NEXT Distro 173

Ni Mhaille, Azzy-Mae 109-116

Nixon, Richard 55

non-judgmental 25, 142, 187, 188, 392, 422

nonaddictive use 285

Nothing About Us Without Us 54

nurse 80, 82, 143

nurturing 371,

nutrition 33, 186, 358,

O

Oakland 83

Offender Treatment Program 225, 230

old-timer 20, 41, 43, 92, 104, 107

one-size-fits-all 13, 91, 92, 130, 142, 169, 177, 200, 268, 301, 415, 420,

one-to-one exchange 89,

opiate use disorder (OUD) 21

opiates 15, 19, 21, 54, 55, 76, 92, 94, 159, 173, 231, 282, 296, 304, 307, 352,

opioid use disorder (OUD) 233

opioids 22, 142, 143, 145, 146, 159, 203, 233, 238, 278, 282, 420

Ousterman, Susan 9, 18, 418-422

outcomes 13, 14, 26, 27, 29, 129, 185, 188, 202, 228, 238, 239, 253, 262, 283, 355, 365, 393, 416

outpatient 64, 164, 245, 281, 309

outreach 13, 20, 44, 79, 105, 112, 163, 164, 166, 171, 181, 186, 187, 226, 294, 295, 297, 346, 440

Over the Influence 63, 302, 383

overdose 9, 10, 11, 22, 42, 54, 55, 82, 90, 110, 112, 119, 126, 130, 157, 159, 169, 173, 174, 177, 183, 189, 192, 203, 204, 213, 250, 282, 295, 297, 298, 302, 303, 304, 352, 353, 354, 398, 410, 420, 422, 428, 443

Overdose Awareness Day 9, 250

overdose prevention centers. See safe consumption sites

OxyContin 233, 234

P

pain 11, 51, 89, 99, 101, 107, 148, 173, 178, 199, 235, 244, 281, 282, 284, 285, 287, 290, 307, 313, 321, 324, 325, 367, 381, 382, 394, 411, 416, 437, 438, 439

pain medication 42, 293

pain patients 55, 282

paranoid 65, 411

paraphernalia 226

parents 9, 10, 49, 94, 96, 118, 163, 164, 165, 176, 188, 239, 257, 261, 305, 306, 319, 320, 353, 366, 367, 377, 378, 387, 388, 389, 391, 393, 394, 399, 418, 419, 420, 421, 427, 429, 432

Park, Albie 307-314

Parks, George 317-329

parole 276,

Parry, Allan 49, 345, 346

partner 10, 13, 82, 101, 106, 133, 192, 193, 281, 287, 326, 360, 366, 374, 378, 383, 400, 402, 405, 406, 407, 409, 411, 429, 437

party drugs 140, 142, 145

pathologizing 193, 284, 445

Peele, Stanton 303, 324, 339, 340

peer pressure 94

peers 42, 64, 104, 140, 141, 184, 195, 249, 273, 296, 297, 299, 328, 425

Peller, Jane 363, 374

people of color 47

Percocet 99, 101

Perls, Fritz 286

Perry, Meghann 15, 424-440

Perry-Stewart, Sophie 424-440

personality disorders 286

peyote 201

pharmaceuticals 378

pharmacology 37

physiological dependence 282

pipes 183, 431

pimps 165

Plymouth 182, 183, 188

Poellot, Erica 191-195

police 40, 44, 82, 101, 104, 144, 158, 260, 346, 412, 413

policy. See drug policy

politicians 82, 399

poor 57, 79, 86, 143, 209, 236, 239, 259, 319, 354

Portland 425

positive change 13, 15, 19, 21, 26, 41, 42, 57, 114, 120, 179, 193, 199, 217, 222, 229, 254, 282, 284, 332, 348, 368, 391, 393, 398

pothead 329

poverty 25, 48, 186, 422

power dynamic

powerlessness

Practicing Harm Reduction Psychotherapy

pragmatism 15, 26, 36, 43, 231, 248, 318, 327, 329

prescribed medication 107, 175,

prevention 33, 159, 163, 166, 173, 183, 192, 245, 246, 294, 295, 300, 322, 323, 325, 326, 327

Prillwitz, Jeremy 331-337

Principles of Harm Reduction 24, 25

prison 72, 181, 185, 186, 292, 326, 372, 402, 413, 438, 442, 444

problematic 11, 23, 40, 52, 114, 116, 118, 142, 203, 204, 210, 244,

281, 284, 285, 287, 289, 292, 356, 357, 363, 366, 383, 396, 420, 427, 432, 433, 435, 437, 439

process addictions 255

prodependency 375

professionalization 144, 145

progressive 37, 47, 249

prohibition 34, 139, 140, 156, 168

prostitute 94, 397

psilocybin 201, 320

psych meds 92, 174

psychedelic 142, 253,

psychiatric 95, 151, 260, 302

psychodrama 286,

psychologist 18, 20, 46, 243, 251, 254, 283, 301, 303, 324, 328

psychology 43, 122, 155, 222, 253, 273, 274, 305, 315, 317, 320, 321, 324, 326, 375

psychosis 260

psychotherapy. See harm reduction psychotherapy

psychotic 149, 260

PTSD 260, 319

public health 53, 83, 109, 110, 111, 146, 200, 212, 225, 231, 302, 311, 312, 313, 318, 327

Puerto Rican 47, 48, 79

punishment 11, 33, 87, 103, 178, 218, 236, 372, 374

punk rock 181, 187

Purchase, Dave 126

PWUD 25, 28, 29, 31, 35, 36, 39, 40,

42, 54, 61, 80, 329

Q

queer 48, 57, 79, 86, 115, 203, 208, 209, 213

R

race 149, 155, 166, 329,

racial justice 82

racism 25, 54, 59, 82, 121, 122, 155, 156, 176, 186, 201, 213, 399

radical 47, 159, 194, 211, 254, 255, 328, 329

rape 95, 105

rapport 96, 169, 265

rave 138, 141

Raymond, Daniel 120

recovery 16, 28, 37, 41, 42, 59, 64, 65, 66, 67, 68, 71, 72, 73, 74, 75, 84, 85, 90, 91, 92, 95, 103, 104, 105, 107, 108, 117, 119, 122, 124, 129, 130, 131, 132, 133, 134, 135, 147, 148, 150, 154, 156, 157, 160, 168, 169, 173, 174, 177, 182, 184, 185, 186, 187, 188, 189, 191, 197, 200, 201, 202, 230, 235, 250, 257, 267, 268, 269, 271, 278, 279, 281, 285, 294, 296, 297, 299, 301, 307, 308, 310, 318, 331, 332, 334, 335, 339, 340, 342, 346, 354, 355, 357, 362, 366, 383, 391, 393, 402, 404, 406, 409, 411, 412, 413, 414, 415, 416, 426, 429, 431, 432, 437, 440

Recovery High School 427

recreational 427, 442

Refuge Recovery 184

regulation 143, 286

rehab 72, 73, 74, 90, 94, 153, 154, 155, 178, 230, 301, 312, 353, 358, 359, 399, 439, 443

Reiki 184

Reiman, Amanda 305

relapse 27, 68, 93, 104, 108, 154, 327, 404, 411, 412, 414

relapse prevention 245, 246, 325, 326, 327

Relapse Prevention (book) 27, 43

relationships 15, 29, 32, 34, 35, 86, 94, 96, 106, 165, 166, 191, 192, 193, 194, 198, 204, 210, 239, 245, 248, 255, 259, 260, 263, 264, 275, 285, 295, 355, 356, 368, 373, 375, 382, 391, 401, 402, 403, 405, 428, 432, 433, 437, 438

Remedy Alliance 226

residential 166, 226, 228, 276, 301, 302, 305, 307, 309, 356, 357

respect 21, 22, 56, 125, 143, 146, 164, 188, 208, 230, 231, 254, 255, 284, 306, 311, 336, 342, 383, 391, 443

Reynolds, Tessa 197-205

Rhoads, Zach 339-343

risk-to-benefit 142

rocks 118, 219

Rodgers, Everett 277

Rogers, Carl 229, 264, 336

Rollnick, Stephen 43, 236, 239, 275

Ross, Alessandra 83

Rosser, Ashley 105

ROTC 319, 320

Rucker, Joy 53

runaways 95, 137, 140, 165

S

Sabora, Chad 117-127

sacrifice 81,

safe consumption sites 159, 170, 204, 329, 422, 435, 440

safe injection facilities. See safe consumption sites

safe supply 19, 140, 143

safer sex 148, 183,

safety 14, 34, 65, 94, 116, 142, 169, 188, 415, 419, 420, 430, 431

safety net 82

safety profile 142

Sage Project 90

Salvation Army 95

SAMHSA 37

San Francisco 20, 39, 63, 71, 75, 79, 80, 89, 90, 95, 181, 182, 228, 230, 231, 308, 312, 328,

San Francisco AIDS Foundation 64, 67

San Francisco Behavioral Health Commission 130

San Francisco Drug Users Union 231

San Jose 84, 186

Sanders, Njon 129-135

Satir, Virginia 371

Scared Straight 94

schizophrenia 260

science 18, 36, 55, 106, 115, 306, 317, 323, 375

science denial 114

Seattle 13, 41, 43, 49, 58, 90, 250, 273, 328

self-care 437, 439

self-destructive 165, 311, 343

self-directed 37, 193, 286, 333

self-disclosure 335

self-esteem 168, 259, 270,

self-hatred 284, 287, 406

self-medication 93

selfish 434

selfless 16, 80, 81

Serenity Prayer 416

sex industry 91,

sex work 86, 90, 91, 112, 121, 165

SF Heroin Committee 90

Sferios, Emanuel 137-146

shaman 415

shame 27, 44, 108, 179, 194, 198, 199, 201, 202, 207, 210, 257, 289, 327, 340, 347, 357, 398, 400, 402, 403, 404, 405, 406

shelter 77, 108, 199, 439

shun 108,

sickle cell anemia 51

Siever, Michael 308, 333, 336

sleep 63, 65, 98, 99, 218, 223, 248, 259, 346, 353, 398, 399, 402, 430

SMART Recovery 104, 278

smoking 107, 175, 187, 315, 354, 425, 431

sober 90, 91, 92, 93, 95, 107, 132, 134, 185, 189, 192, 201, 202, 238, 239, 245, 250, 268, 331, 364, 391, 395, 396, 402, 404, 409, 410, 433

sober-curious 23

sober house 105, 107, 181

sobriety 107, 130, 165, 174, 184, 218, 237, 240, 247, 250, 308, 310, 311, 402, 409, 410, 411, 412, 420

social justice 21, 23, 41, 80, 121

social services 422

social support 37

social worker 80, 82, 269, 305, 328, 345

socialist 80, 218, 220,

socioeconomic 120

soup kitchen 75

South Bronx 48

speed balls 187

spirituality 37, 358

sponsor 66, 74, 102, 105, 114, 132, 177, 244, 267, 331, 358, 414

Springer, Edith 49, 83, 120, 345-348

SSI 79, 80, 294

St. Paul 220

stabilization 250, 285, 397

Stages of Change 310, 315, 364

Stancliff, Sharon 193

STDs 63, 112

stealing 101, 187, 319

Steil, Chris 147-151

Stella Maris 102, 103

sterile 95, 165, 192, 421, 436

Stiers, David Ogden 351

stigma 79, 86, 94, 105, 106, 108, 110, 127, 142, 143, 146, 179, 182, 194, 198, 201, 203, 205, 255, 267, 270, 304, 305, 318, 329, 348, 402, 418, 420, 421, 442, 443

Stimulant Treatment Outpatient Program (STOP) 309

stimulants 92, 145, 278

stinking thinking 132,

Stonewall Project 64, 308, 309, 310, 333,

Stout, Dee-Dee 331, 377

strategy 21, 22, 25, 36, 41, 43, 85, 94, 131, 177, 184, 192, 197, 210, 233, 251, 257, 263, 274, 284, 296, 297, 298, 321, 328, 332, 354, 355, 359, 375, 391, 393, 394, 427, 434, 437, 443

stress 24, 51, 178, 186, 234, 286, 365, 378, 391, 394, 399

Suboxone 93, 103, 173, 174, 226, 231, 442, 443

Substance Abuse and Mental Health Services Administration (SAMHSA) 37

substance use 10, 14, 15, 34, 38, 86, 105, 163, 164, 168, 192, 193, 198, 200, 202, 203, 205, 233, 245, 246, 247, 250, 254, 263, 269, 281, 284, 285, 286, 288, 289, 292, 295, 301, 302, 304, 308, 313, 332, 335, 336, 356, 379, 391, 392, 418, 419, 420,

421, 422, 425, 426, 429, 432, 436

substance use disorder (SUD) 10, 14, 15, 26, 36, 37, 38, 55, 126, 127, 165, 166, 175, 178, 191, 192, 227, 243, 246, 250, 261, 267

suffering 52, 154, 186, 187, 262, 284, 285, 287, 321, 329, 381, 402, 405, 418, 429, 436, 437

suicide 174, 301, 396, 414

support group 15, 39, 132, 222, 358, 376

surrender 393

survival sex 91

Sweden 346

symptom 34, 51, 148, 259, 373, 375, 376, 378, 420

syringe 15, 67, 89, 95, 110, 111, 112, 124, 154, 159, 167, 169, 179, 192, 208, 293, 294, 296, 297, 298, 299, 300, 411, 421, 425, 444

syringe services programs (SSPs) 19, 83, 163, 166, 167, 182, 183, 184, 188, 192, 249, 299

Szalavitz, Maia 18, 153-161

Szyler, John 42

T

Tapestry Needle Exchange 208

Tatarsky, Andrew 20, 283, 289, 303, 328

Taughinbaugh, Cathy 391-394

teens 45, 46, 90, 137, 138, 140, 165, 208, 257, 339, 388, 389, 427, 428, 432

Tenderloin 79, 96, 187, 226, 227,

231

Tennessee 176

Thatcher, Margaret 346

THC 199

the rooms 68, 77, 175, 177, 191, 410, 416

therapeutic boarding school 395

therapeutic community (TC) 102

third person 289

thirteenth step 113

Thrive Behavioral Health 104

Tik-Tok 97

Tilley, Jess 207-214

tobacco 11, 354

tolerance 157, 188, 406

tough love 94, 178, 301, 311, 313, 335, 354, 357, 371, 373, 380, 381, 382

tracks 64, 66, 411

trafficking 438

Train the Trainers (ToT) 83

training 20, 25, 37, 46, 49, 54, 83, 84, 85, 112, 123, 125, 166, 210, 233, 234, 243, 245, 253, 255, 263, 265, 274, 275, 276, 277, 305, 322, 326, 333, 335, 346, 361, 362, 374, 388, 422

trans 79, 86, 91, 95, 112, 115

transition 97, 111, 245, 268, 332, 401

trap-house 101

trauma 25, 34, 98, 138, 160, 198, 202, 205, 208, 210, 225, 228, 230, 234, 270, 282, 284, 286, 287, 289,

292, 301, 319, 335, 363, 373, 376, 395, 396, 407, 420, 422, 432, 438, 444

treatment centers 91, 102, 104, 154, 177, 178, 281, 326, 328, 362, 374

trigger 32, 66, 274, 403

Trimingham, Tony 380

trust 24, 42, 50, 168, 173, 227, 239, 264, 306, 364, 365, 380, 398, 426, 431, 443

Tula, Monique 53, 208

tweaker 67

12 Step 14, 32, 36, 39, 40, 42, 43, 44, 48, 65, 66, 68, 69, 72, 73, 74, 75, 77, 93, 94, 97, 105, 107, 110, 112, 113, 119, 124, 131, 132, 133, 147, 148, 150, 154, 174, 175, 177, 184, 185, 191, 192, 193, 202, 209, 218, 237, 243, 244, 245, 248, 251, 263, 267, 268, 270, 271, 280, 281, 311, 318, 320, 331, 332, 334, 335, 345, 347, 356, 401, 409, 416, 427, 428, 430

U

UCLA 279

unconditional positive regard 202, 256

unethical 35, 141

unhoused 82, 83, 86, 140, 201, 202

unjust laws 337

University of Washington 13, 43, 250, 273, 320

urine test 198

V

Vakharia, Sheila 303

vegetarian 187

Veterans' Drug Treatment Court 102

Vilomah Foundation 9

violence 52, 86, 95, 165

Violette, Lorie 163-170

voice 12, 25, 53, 135, 159, 194, 286, 287, 288, 290, 359, 402, 403

Volkow, Nora 10

voluntary 114

volunteer 90, 115, 133, 137, 141, 163, 164, 167, 209, 221, 261, 268, 273, 294

vulnerability 25, 407

W

Walden House 92

War on Drugs 11, 15, 21, 40, 41, 55, 82, 124, 137, 155, 176, 201, 211, 270, 282, 302, 304, 318, 399, 418

Ward 86 80

water 19, 65, 90, 95, 129, 187, 201, 419, 426

weed 66, 76, 139, 189, 347, 389, 402, 424, 425, 426, 427, 430, 431, 432, 433

Wegscheider-Cruse, Sharon 356

Weil, Andrew 324

welfare 72, 239, 294, 362

wellness 28, 37, 114, 131, 173, 270, 323, 327, 375, 383

Wheeler, Eliza 112, 120, 226

White 45, 46, 49, 51, 52, 53, 54, 56, 57, 84, 119, 156, 213, 264, 351, 356, 399

white knuckling 132

wife 73, 75, 77, 105, 269, 293, 356

Wilson, Bill 220, 356, 358

Wilson, Lois 356

wine 76, 274, 313, 377

withdrawal 91, 158, 220, 226, 444

Woods, Imani 48, 56, 58

X

Xanax 352

xenophobia 122

Y

yoga 184, 187,

Young Lords Organization (YLO) 47

youth 47, 80, 95, 97, 166, 226

Z

Zane, Brenda 387-389

zealotry 122